MY BROTHER CANCER

Helen and Leonard Bee
the story of an unbreakable bond

*What you need to know to manage the disease
and your oncologist*

by Adele Bianchi and Parisio Di Giovanni

you ought to know

Title: My brother cancer.
What you need to know to manage the disease
and your oncologist

Authors: Adele Bianchi and Parisio Di Giovanni

On the cover: «On the hill», oil painting on canvas
by Eugenio and Parisio Di Giovanni

translated with the collaboration of Rosie Trachtman

ISBN-13: 978-1517661014

ISBN-10: 1517661013

Introduction

When cancer comes into your life, because you or someone close to you gets sick, you become upset. You tend to think that things have changed radically. Sometimes people go so far as to no longer consider life really life: the patient has the impression that his life is over even though it's still going on, and others look at him as one who is alive but no longer is alive.

What distorts your thoughts is the positivity bias, also known as the Pollyanna principle or Pollyannaism, terms derived from the name of the protagonist of the famous novel by Eleanor Porter. People tend to think positive events more frequent and more likely than negative ones. Therefore, normal life seems to be made of health, well-being, success and justice, while diseases, hardships, failures and injustices are exceptions.

The positivity bias is useful, since it drives people to face life with confidence and commitment. But it provides a false impression of life. People don't realize how this really is. So, when misfortune comes, they are unprepared and make mistakes.

Statistics can open our eyes. The latest available say that about 15 million people in the world every year are diagnosed with cancer, on average about 2 per 1,000 people. The data varies from across the world. In a country like the United States in one year about 5 per 1,000 people became ill with cancer and about 2 of 1,000 have died from this disease. According to these data, in the United States, people who are lucky enough to live a long life-span have a more than one in three chance of getting cancer, the lifetime probability of developing the disease is 43.3% for men and 37.8 for women. Among other things, cancer is increasing and these probabilities will be higher in the coming years. It is clear that cancer is widely present in our lives and we should reasonably expect it to occur, either that we get sick or someone close to us becomes ill.

Once diagnosed, the cancer remains with you as long as you live, either the disease continues to reoccur after a period of silence, or it leaves you to the end, afraid of its return. Cancer is now part of your life. Helen, the protagonist of the story told in the book, says this suggestively when she calls her cancer "my brother cancer." Therefore it makes little sense to look at life with new eyes, to not consider it life anymore, just because a cancer appeared. This is the first robust teaching that the book contains: life with cancer is fully life. If you leave behind the Pollyannaism and understand this key point, it will be easier for you to accept this fact: cancer is a chronic disease. Especially if the cancer is metastatic, the important thing is to keep it at bay not delete it. If you go on to live and live well, the care is perfect, even if the cancer is in your body. Considering cancer an acute illness is an error, which causes you to exceed with the treatments or, conversely, to surrender.

Here's another important lesson that you can find in Helen and Leonard's story: you have to manage cancer as a chronic disease. Medicine is committed to finding weapons to fight cancer. Perhaps one day we will succeed, as happened with other diseases that also claimed victims. But you get sick now and can only rely on what medicine has discovered so far. For you the most important thing is not to go looking for miraculous remedies, but how to cope with your illness in the best way possible with the means we have today, living for as long as possible and in the best possible conditions. Managing cancer is an art, which requires sophisticated knowledge, reasoning and philosophy.

The story of Helen, who manages her disease with the help of her husband Leonard, an eclectic and unusual doctor, allows us to understand many key points in the management of cancer. There is also the problem of managing oncologists, who for a number of reasons sometimes are not the best advisors.

The first part of the book tells the story of Helen and Leonard struggling with this " problematic brother". Helen's is an "amazing case", as defined by a famous physician and researcher in touch with Leonard. It is particular not only for the success of the treatment, but also for how they decide to do things, for the rationality, wisdom and courage that Helen and Leonard show in making decisions together.

In the events of this story of cancer nestle many lessons for anyone who wants to better manage the disease and oncologists. In the second part of the book some of these lessons are illustrated neatly. The story of Helen and Leonard and perhaps this book can help those suffering from the disease, their loved ones, but also doctors, health workers and all of us.

Adele Bianchi and Parisio Di Giovanni

Contents

*Leonard and Helen's adventure
in struggling with cancer*

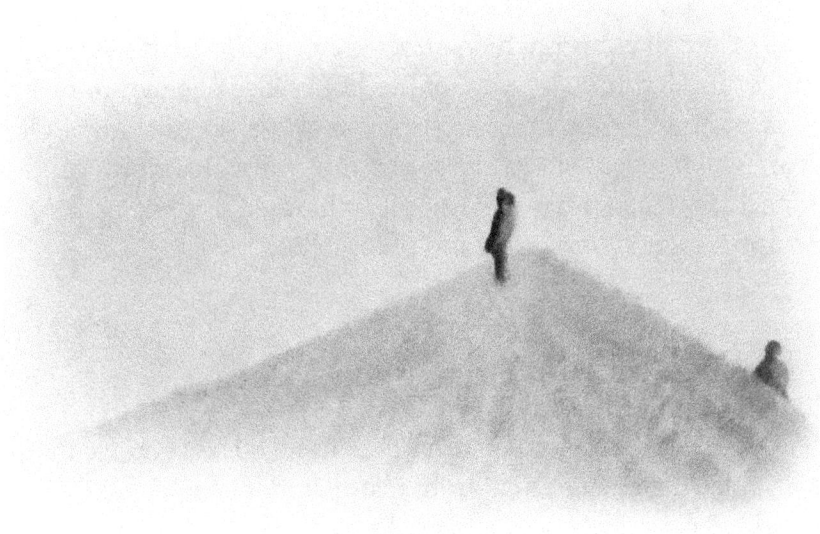

Cancer shows up in Helen's life

There are twenty days left until her fifty-fifth birthday, which falls on Christmas day, when Helen discovers that she has a cancer, which is already very advanced. She is a psychologist, and together with her husband Leonard who is a doctor and university professor, she is teaching a training course for doctors. At one point Leonard and some other doctors who are taking the course look at her from afar, carefully and with a strange clinical look on their faces; her husband comes up to her and says "Your abdomen is swelled up, it seems like you have ascites, an abdominal accumulation of fluid, we have to have examinations done, I've already made the appointments for tomorrow".

At home later that evening, her husband examines her, and determined that there is liquid in her abdomen. The next day, ultrasound and CT scan show that in addition to the ascites, she had diffuse visceral cancer, which affected her peritoneum, stomach, ovaries, and left ureter. Some of her bones also seemed to be affected by the disease. A gastroscopy shows a serious linitis plastica, which is a widespread cancerous involvement of the stomach, in which the wall is entirely infiltrated by neoplastic cells and appears rigid, wrinkled and deformed.

But it was already there

All of a sudden certain disturbances that she has had for many years, and that they had all underestimated, become clear. Over time, Helen had been loosing a lot of weight, she sometimes threw up after meals, at night she has had heartburn, and her ankles tended to swell. She had taken some medical tests, but hadn't found anything of importance.

If truth must be told, a few things which could have helped point to the right diagnosis had emerged. In a gastroscopy that she had taken the year before, her stomach had appeared somewhat rigid. It had seemed to the specialist like a simple motility disturbance, seeing as how the mucosa was healthy, and as seen from the inside, the stomach seemed healthy. Leonard had theorized that the rigidity could have been caused by a tumor that may have infiltrated the external layers of the stomach wall, and which for that reason, couldn't be seen from the inside. But the specialist, had dismissed his idea as the fetched hypothesis of a worried husband, "What could you possibly be thinking!". Leonard had let himself be convinced to think positively. We all very much like to believe that everything is going well and ignore the warning signs!

Two years earlier an ultrasound examination of her abdomen had revealed a slight stricture of the left ureter, the canal which brings urine from the kidney to the bladder. Leonard and the ecographist hadn't thought that it was particularly important. Two years later, with the illness in full force, Leonard discovered that the ureter, specifically on the left side, is typically one of the first sites involved by the metastatic cancer that his wife was now suffering from.

Leonard goes back to being a doctor

It is now clear that she has metastatic cancer. But what kind of cancer is it? Where did it start? And what might be the best way to deal with it? Leonard is much too overwrought to think as a doctor about his own wife's illness. The thing that haunts him most is his sense of guilt. In hindsight he torments himself with the realization that he could have, and should have been able to detect the disease much earlier, at a stage where it would have been much easier to treat. Helen, on the other hand, is calm and distant, it is as if she is looking in on somebody else's illness story. Therefore she is the one who supports Leonard, and trying to make things easier, she encourages him to give the responsibility of her care to a highly skilled specialist.

They go to a center of excellence where, after examining Helen, the specialist calls Leonard to the side and passes a strong sentence: this is an ovarian cancer, very advanced, I'm not sure if we should start chemotherapy, because I believe that your wife does not have three months to live.

Pushed by desperation, they act on the advice of a relative who is a pathologist, and approach a famous oncologist Stephen T., who is more possibilist: it could be ovarian cancer, but it could also possibly be gastric, or even breast cancer, and we must attempted a treatment that could be effective in all three cases. He considers among others, the possibility of mammary origin because he has in the past seen cases of breast cancer with similar patterns of metastatic spread. Unlike the other specialist, this one seems cautiously hopeful and recommends chemotherapy using docetaxel + capecitabine.

In the meantime, Helen's condition has been rapidly worsening. She has lost a lot of weight, doesn't eat and is very weak, all signs of cancer cachexia, a syndrome that usually suggests that the tumor is prevailing over the organism and that the end might be coming closer. Helen is checked into the hospital for chemotherapy, as an inpatient her condition can be constantly monitored and she can be given all of the supportive care that she needs.

Over Helen's time in the hospital, Leonard realizes that in fact, they are not capable of giving his wife all of the care that she actually needs. She should be on a special diet for her cachexia, her water balance should be being monitored (by measuring urine and fluid intake), her electrolytes should be kept at normal levels, especially the potassium, which tends to drop to dangerous levels, which can lead to heart disease, sometimes fatal. Leonard tries to talk with his physician colleagues who work in the department, they justify themselves telling him that such a high level of care could be given only in an intensive care unit. The doctors politely try to make him understand that in any case the whole treatment is useless because his wife is dieing of cancer. The oldest doctor invites him to his office and closes the door, he comes up to him and quietly tells him, "Maybe you haven't yet understood, but it is all over, your love seems to be making you blind."

At this point, Leonard has an abrupt wake up call. He resolves to devote himself with all of his strength to Helen's recovery. He will not think about the past any more, but devote himself to the challenge in front of him, the one challenge that to the others seems to be already lost. The thing that really shakes him up is a recurring voice in his head that keeps on asking him: how is it possible that a doctor gives up so easily to cancer, to the point that they stop taking care of other simpler problems, and let a patient die from other causes.

He brings his wife home, and organizes to devote himself night and day to her care. Seeing as how Helen is unable to feed herself, he puts her under a continuous infusion and feeds her parenterally. He takes daily samples of her blood, and constantly monitors her heart and other vital parameters with a electrocardiograph and other instruments and maintains her hydro-electric balance. He is skilled in this kind of treatment because when he was younger he had spent twenty years working as a geriatrician. He was used to dedicating himself patiently to his work with elderly patients in serious conditions, who had been given up on by other doctors, he had at times been able to make unexpected progress, so much so that he had been given the nickname "get up and walk".

United against the disease

Leonard starts to thoroughly study the cachexia, which he knows little about, and develops careful strategies for Helen's feeding, care and monitoring. He takes into consideration standard procedures, but also follows a personalized plan which he constantly adapts to his wife's specific condition. A little at a time, Helen starts to be able to feed herself, and Leonard prepares a targeted diet, a diet, which is properly balanced and which contains a series of food supplements useful to combat the cachexia. Helen and Leonard meticulously weigh ingredients, measure out supplements, and calculate calories, proteins, fats and sugars and keep daily charts with all of the information. Diligently doing this work Helen and Leonard hope that their commitment will be repaid and above all they feel united, perhaps more than ever before. Blood and urine tests help Leonard adjust the diet to the changing conditions of his wife.

Oncologists with the fixation of going to war against cancer

During the time that he is working to manage his wife's diet, Leonard starts to have serious doubts about the mindset that he encounters in many oncologists. Technicians and doctors in the labs where he sends blood and urine samples are often surprised by the tests that he asks to have done, and ask him what he will do with the information that he gets from them. For example, they ask him why he wants to measure the prealbumin in blood samples, instead of just measuring the albumin, or why he frequently collects 24-hour urine samples to measure their nitrogen levels. They wonder why oncologists don't have these tests done, even though there are plenty of patients in the hospital who, like Helen are suffering from neoplastic cachexia.

The lab technicians and doctors find Leonard's explanations very interesting, so much so that they're careful to record changes of value in the tests that he's taking. They interpret the tests together with him, discovering with satisfaction that they are useful. But why don't more oncologists make use of these exams? Leonard becomes more and more convinced that it is because they don't consider cachexia to be an important enough condition to work carefully on: they are more focused on the cancer itself, than on the nutritional state of the person with cancer.

A famous oncologist offers to give him advice, and while talking with him Leonard becomes further convinced of his idea that oncologists tend to be overly focused on the cancer itself. The oncologist asks him in a reproachful tone why he is giving Helen supplements such as arginine and glutamine when they could "feed the cancer". Leonard, who has read many articles on the topic, knows that in the case of arginine, there is some truth to the concern, whereas it is highly doubtful that glutamine can promote cancer: glutamine seems to have a selective action mechanism which strengthens healthy cells, while at the same time weakening neoplastic ones. There is a question that shakes Leonard's mind: what is the point of letting cachexia destroy the body only to avoid giving a slight advantage to the tumor? If her organism gives up, we've lost Helen. It's true that we have to make things difficult for the tumor, but we must do this in a balanced fashion, without penalizing the organism that we are trying to save.

The diagnosis comes in

Leonard studies tenaciously, and works hard to achieve the diagnosis of origin, and see whether the primary tumor is ovarian, mammary or gastric. He asks a relative of his, who is a pathologist, to carefully examine biopsies taken from her stomach.

While seeing the test results he begins to think that the tumor might have a mammary origin, not gastric or ovarian, as it had seemed to the specialist consulted at the beginning. There is a kind of cell which is known as a signet ring cell. These cancer cells are called this because they are full of mucus and thus looks like rings with a stone set in them. Signet ring cells are typical of stomach cancer, but Helen's cancer can't be gastric. In fact, chemical exams of the neoplastic cells demonstrate that the molecular markers of gastro-intestinal tumors aren't present, instead they find, mammaglobin and GCDFP-15, which are specific markers for mammary cancer. There are also estrogen and progesterone receptors, which even though they direct us more towards mammary cancer, still don't give us certainties because we can find them also in gastric and ovarian cancers.

Moreover, during his studies, Leonard learns that signet ring cells can be present also in mammary cancer. In particular in one type of mammary cancer, the invasive lobular, which has a mucinous variant, which is made of signet ring cells, just like gastric cancer.

At this point, Leonard has become a tireless scholar of scientific literature on the subject: for every question that comes to his mind, he finds on the Internet scientific articles which were published about this issue and systematically reviews them. It is a great help the fact that he has spent a good part of his life studying and doing research, although in other fields and perhaps never so obstinately. Through his research, he discovers an important fact: over the past twenty years, studies have been published which describe clinical cases similar to Helen's which were caused by primitive breast tumors, from which, the cancer spreads to other parts of the body. These primitive tumors are frequently found in the breast only after the cancer has spread to the abdomen, or they aren't found at all, and remain -as they say- hidden. For the most part, oncologists ignore the fact that this can happen, and frequently make mistaken diagnosis. That which Stephen T. had suspected based on his personal clinical experience, has been scientifically documented.

Immediately, Leonard has Helen get radiological exams done in order to find the primitive tumor. Leonard had already carefully palpated the mammary tissue without finding anything. The mammogram and resonance imaging also come back negative, but Leonard knows that primitive tumors, especially if they are lobular invasive, can frequently be occult, that is that they can't be seen with radiographic methods. On the other hand, the mammogram shows the presence of small calcifications, which can sometimes be caused by cancer.

By now, he is convinced that Helen's cancer started in her breast. He still feels the need though , to ask for another opinion from afar, a remote second opinion from a well known specialized breast cancer center. Their response makes him feel more sure. The doctor that writes back to him is also convinced that Helen's metastatic cancer certainly or almost certainly originates from the breast. The expert is nearly certain in her diagnosis, because, in the medical center where she works, they treat a very large number of cases of breast cancer every year, she has had a lot of experience, and has seen cases similar to Helen's.

Still not satisfied, Leonard has another test done on the cells of the stomach biopsy: the study of the estrogen receptor profile. The test that pathologists routinely give, shows only one kind of receptor (the alpha receptor), but research has shown that another kind of receptor also exists (beta receptors). In mammary lobular invasive cancer, the different types of receptors are combined in a characteristic profile. Leonard has trouble finding a pathologist who will do an alpha/beta study, but in the end he finds one, and the profile is that of lobular invasive cancer.

At this point, the diagnosis seems clear. What convinces Leonard isn't only the clinical picture and the various tests that he had done, but also a simple thought process: for women, breast cancer is much more frequent than ovarian or gastric cancers. Leonard is an expert in the field of human reasoning, he has done research on the causes of reasoning errors of doctors and he knows that it is a common mistake to ignore the likelihood that a specific person might have a specific disease, and base the diagnosis only on facts that manifest themselves once the illness is already present. Even if the clinical picture and tests had left us with doubts, the mammary origin would still have been the most likely diagnosis. If we add the fact that the clinical features and tests all point to a mammary cancer, the diagnosis becomes so likely, that we can nearly consider it certain.

After diagnosis, a successful chemotherapy

The diagnosis of the origin is important when choosing a treatment. The chemotherapy recommended by Stephen T. works much better in mammary cancer than in ovarian or gastric cancers. Leonard discusses it with Helen, and together they decide to go with this treatment.

After three cycles of docetaxel and capecitabine, the illness improves, and after six cycles, there is a complete remission, that is, there are no more clinical signs of the disease. The ascites has disappeared, Helen has recovered both her weight and her strength, magnetic resonance and PET-CT scans are normal, and the blood markers which had originally been high have dropped to normal levels (CA 15-3, CA 125, CA 72-4, CEA, ferritin). Nothing more is found with the gastroscopy.

Still dealing with the fixation of going to war against cancer

Certain oncologists recommend another three cycles of therapy, in order to attack the tumor more completely, but in Leonard's opinion, continuing with chemotherapy is foolish. It is true that the disease is still present, even if clinical exams don't permit us to see it any more. There are definitely still some cancerous cells left in various parts of the body which aren't giving signs of their presence, either because they are dormant or inactive, or because they form masses which are too small to be shown by common imaging diagnostic methods. This fact though, does not make it a good idea to continue with chemotherapy.

Chemotherapy, even if highly effective, and with long periods of treatment, will never be able to destroy all of the cancerous cells. Both research, and clinical experience have shown that a certain amount of cancerous cells, whether in large or small numbers, will resist even the most aggressive of therapies and be able to survive. If there is no hope of eradicating her cancer, and eliminating it once and for all, exposing Helen to additional cycles of chemotherapy, would only lead to making her suffer further, and expose her to ulterior risks.

A complete remission is the best possible result, the treatment has already done what it was capable of doing. The important thing now, is that Helen recovers from both the physical damage, and from the hardships that come with six cycles of chemotherapy, and is able to go back to her normal life. Maybe even more important at this point, is not to let her be exposed to any further risks.

Double edged swords to manage with care

Chemotherapy is dangerous: if cancer weren't the terrible disease that it is, we wouldn't even think of treating people with such fearsome treatments. During these first six cycles, Helen and Leonard had experienced one of the tremendous dangers that come with this type of treatment. Her third infusion of docetaxel had been going for a few minutes, when Helen suddenly had a feeling of chest tightness, she had difficulty breathing and was quickly becoming pale. "I thought that I was going to die" she later explained. Leonard immediately stopped the infusion: which is the first thing that should be done in these cases. It seemed very much like a type 1 hypersensitivity reaction, a reaction that can be caused by docetaxel, especially after the second infusion.

Luckily, within a few minutes, Helen had gotten back to herself. She was already in better condition when a doctor and a nurse arrived, recalled by the alarm that Leonard had rung right after stopping the infusion. The nurse, to Leonard's great surprise, had put a basin to vomit into on Helen's belly, even though she hadn't shown any sign of nausea, and docetaxel isn't among the chemotherapy drugs that usually stimulate vomiting. The doctor had noticed that the infusion had been stopped, and resentfully nearly threatened Leonard: how dare you do something like that?

Once the moment of turmoil had passed, and the doctor seemed to have calmed down somewhat, Leonard explained to her that there had been hypersensitivity symptoms, and that immediately stopping the infusion, frequently makes these symptoms disappear within a few minutes.

With these clarifications, the psychological climate returned to an acceptable level. In any case, Helen kept repeating that she still wasn't sure about wanting to do chemotherapy, and Leonard was objectively worried. A hypersensitivity reaction can cause death, and the department didn't seem to be prepared to manage certain risks. Among other things, the doctors and nurses had seemed doubtful and hesitant when Leonard told them that from now on they could only continue giving her docetaxel, if they agreed to go very slowly, and to put a pulse oximeter on her finger to measure her vital signs.

Someone objected that prolonging treatment time was problematic in a day hospital, open from eight in the morning till two in the afternoon. Others worried that seeing Helen with the pulse oximeter on her finger would push other patients to complain and ask for the same level of attention to their care. Leonard was shocked: a pulse oximeter should always be used when administering chemotherapy, even more so with someone who has already had a negative reaction to the treatment, moreover, lengthening infusion times is the rule, even if there is only a suspect of a hypersensitivity reaction. He hadn't been expecting such a careless attitude, especially after all the cases of fatal administration of chemotherapy made famous by the media, and the publication of scientific statistics about accidents in this field and the subsequent detailed recommendations on risk management.

Leonard was a university professor who enjoyed prestige and familiarity in the medical world. He spoke with the director of the oncology department, and that of the intensive care unit. He asked for and obtained an agreement that Helen's infusions from then on would be held in an adequate department, with the correct precautions, and under his direct supervision. Helen felt reassured, and under these conditions agreed to continue the chemotherapy: a good thing, because it all went for the best. But would the story have ended differently had Leonard not been there to interrupt the infusion? And had he been unable to make sure that Helen's chemotherapy be done as it should be? In the coming years Helen and Leonard would frequently return to ask themselves these questions.

No, doing another three sessions of chemotherapy did not make sense. In the beginning, it had been a desperate situation, the cancer had been killing Helen. For this reason it had been worth the risk, the chemotherapy was justified. Continuing it after having obtained results though, meant foolishly playing with destiny: Helen would be exposed for another three cycles to all the dangers that she had been lucky to survive during the first six cycles, without any good reason, because in any case we can be sure that some cancer cells would survive in her body.

Helen switches to hormone therapy and Leonard studies and meditates about certain oddities of medicine

There are still some cancer cells in Helen's body, for this reason even if it is a bad idea to continue with chemotherapy, waiting and doing nothing is a mistake. Luckily, Helen's cancer can be treated with hormone therapy, which can be done from the comfort of their own home, is well tolerated, and doesn't present the risks of chemotherapy. Hormonal therapies do not slaughter cancer cells, as well as a chemotherapy does when it works, but they can keep the cancer cells at bay (slow their growth, keep them dormant, kill some of them). In this way hormonal therapies prevent the disease from coming back, or at least somewhat slow down the disease's revival: an ideal response in this moment of peace.

Not all kinds of breast cancers respond to hormone therapy. Helen's should respond though, because the neoplastic cells have estrogen receptors, through which, in multiple ways the hormonal treatment usually does its job. In Helen's case, there are two other things that suggest that hormone therapy should work: the cells also have progesterone receptors in addition to an adequate amount of beta estrogen receptors. The latter are not routinely assessed, but Leonard has them analyzed in order to be sure of the diagnosis of origin.

Among the things that Leonard has learned in his studies about hormone therapy, there is one aspect which even though it is not important in Helen's case, is of specific interest to him, thinking of all the cases in which it could be of particular help. In clinical practice, the decision of whether or not to use hormone therapy, is based on the presence of alpha receptors, the only receptors to be routinely examined. If the alpha receptor test is positive, the hormone therapy is used, if not, it is taken for granted that hormone therapy doesn't work with that type of tumor, and chemotherapy is considered the only possible option. However the research done over the last few years demonstrates that even tumors which test negatively for alpha receptors can respond to hormone therapy in the presence of a specific kind of beta receptor, called beta 1.

One day, Leonard visits his pathologist relative who had helped him from the beginning, bringing with him a scientific publication which begins polemically: every year, many women who suffer from breast cancer are made to undergo perfectly avoidable chemotherapy by oncologists. The pathologist starts to read the article, turns pale, goes back to reading, and says: a lot of time passes before research gets transferred to clinical practice, because the new information has to become widely known, and the new practices need to become well established, before doctors take responsibility for non standard clinical decisions.

It's true - thought Leonard - it's understandable and altogether human, but if in the meantime many women are denied the advantages of hormone therapy, there is something which isn't working.

Helen's cancer has estrogen receptors, of the alpha type, those which are usually considered for deciding whether or not to use hormone therapy, we are within the norm. In any case, Leonard knows that the presence of these receptors doesn't give us a 100% assurance that the therapy will work. In around 40% of cases, the receptors are there, but the therapy is unsuccessful, probably either because the receptors don't work, or because they aren't important for the cancer cell's growth. There is a way to be certain, but it requires two PET scans, one before and the other after taking estrogen pills for a day. This test isn't usually done in clinical practice, but Leonard knows someone who is willing to perform it. There's a problem though: Helen's PET scan is completely negative, a wonderful fact, which means that if there are neoplastic lesions, they are very small, under 4-5 millimeters. Seeing as how for the test we need to measure at least one lesion both before and after taking the estrogen pill, Leonard has to do without this information, which would have given him more certainty.

After careful study and thought, Leonard decides to use tamoxifen. It is a classic hormone therapy which for multiple reasons should work well against Helen's tumor. The reasons are based on advanced research (for example, the ratio of alpha receptors and various types of beta receptors) which oncologists don't usually pay attention to when making decisions, and which don't give him complete certainty. But Leonard's thought processes was that when we have to try something, being without certainties, clues are always welcome and it is a good idea to use all of the information we can gather, although the uncertainty is still with us despite our best efforts.

Studying about tamoxifen, Leonard discovers a fact which he, as a researcher who studies errors of judgment that doctors make, finds particularly interesting. The history of this drug is a good example of how we tend to mistakenly understand the likelihood that a particular event will come to pass, if the event is emotionally charged, if it bothers us to imagine it. Statistics published in the nineties had caused alarm: tamoxifen can provoke second tumors in the uterus or gastrointestinal tract. Prescriptions dropped low enough that the World Health Organization and the International Agency for Cancer research, intervened to make it clear that there was no reason to deny women the benefits of a drug like tamoxifen. The risk was actually objectively low, especially thinking about the lost benefit caused by avoiding the treatment, but it seemed larger than it was because the thought of a second cancer scares us.

It's extremely difficult to manage our thoughts when it comes to taking risks! At one time a doctor is ready to subject the patient to serious risks with more cycles of chemotherapy in the illusion of winning a war which he can't actually win. Another time he lacks the courage to expose the patient to a small risk, despite the benefit that his actions most likely will bring. Leonard imposes on himself to manage his thoughts and starts with tamoxifen therapy.

Relaxing, yet being on guard so as not to be taken by surprise

During a ceasefire, one can take advantage of the inactivity in order to dedicate time and energy to oneself, regain balance in life, and find a trajectory. Helen and Leonard buy a new car, which would end up being useful, because they will have to travel a lot later on. They go to Venice, and spend ten days in a fancy hotel, with a private dock where a rented motorboat passes by to pick them up to tour and look around. Always having been moderate, they had never indulged in such folly before, which they were now doing with a sort of interior moderation, paying tribute to life. Their son and his girlfriend met them in Venice, and together they continued to tour and look around, reflecting about the gift of life, and about love.

It was only a ceasefire though: sooner or later the cancer would be back to threaten them. It was therefore necessary to plan the tests. The oncologists advised them to measure the tumor markers every 30 - 40 days, and the PET-CT scan first at three months, and then, if the test results were negative, to repeat them every 6-7 months, and, if it seems to be the case, reduce them even more over time. This plan doesn't convince Leonard. To start with, the PET-CT scan should be done every few months.

It seemed to him that a simple thought process was enough to show that 6-7 months between one PET-CT scan and the next was too long. Tumors grow and spread exponentially. As long as a mass of cells is small, under 1 or 2 millimeters, it can remain stable for a long time, as if it is resting, or at the most, grow slowly. After that threshold though, mechanisms are activated which increasingly accelerate the growth: the cells wake up and escape the control of the immune system, they invade the surrounding tissues more easily, and they can feed and discharge waste, using new vessels, created with an activity called tumoral angiogenesis. The cells, still using these new vessels, can migrate and implant themselves elsewhere. For this reason, a slow growth after a certain point, becomes an avalanche.

The PET-CT scan, has a resolution power of 4-5 millimeters, that means that it can't show lesions which are smaller than that size. It can thus happen that today the test comes back negative, but there are already small masses of 1 or 2 millimeters or more. The avalanche, the process of tumor progression which continually increases in speed, has already started but the PET-CT scan doesn't register anything new. If unfortunately this is the situation and we wait 6-7 months, we run the risk of finding ourselves suddenly having to deal with a dramatic picture of having jumped from a silent illness, to an advanced one.

Sometimes oncologists believe that it's better to avoid the PET-CT scan, because the radiation that it produces can be harmful. At times they also have another way of thinking: if the illness reappears, we will have to do chemotherapy, using chemotherapy is justified only if the illness is advanced enough, so it's better to wait.

It didn't make much sense to Leonard to accept the threat that the cancer could devastate the organism, just because of concerns about radiation effects: in a person who is sick with metastatic cancer the first risk (being killed by the cancer) far outweighs the second (suffering damages from the radiation), it's like staying in a collapsing house during an earthquake because of a fear of burglars. The reasoning about the chemotherapy, in his opinion, needed to be overturned and replaced with another, more possibilist and creative way of thinking: chemotherapy should be used if the illness is already in an advanced stage, however if we discover it earlier, we then have the possibility to act on time, we can find other less aggressive methods to manage and treat it.

Precisely because he considered an early discovery of a comeback of the illness useful, he tended to repeat frequently the marker tests, around once every 15 days. He wanted to carefully study their trends, so he put all the results into graphs, fully aware - as an expert in the field - that our minds are easily tricked and don't always notice changes that occur over time if we don't have the help of graphs and we have to rely on our memories and numeral comparisons. He knew that biochemical progression, the increase of markers, frequently precedes the clinical progression of the illness and can be used as an alarm signal.

For the same reason, because he wanted to be ahead of the game, Leonard considered gastroscopies for monitoring the disease, to be very important. The stomach had been completely invaded by the tumor, and it was likely that it would reappear in the same place. The peritoneum had also been largely affected, but looking at the stomach is much easier: it's enough to do a simple clinical exam, the gastroscopy. To those that told him that he should be satisfied with the PET-CT exams, he answered that a gastroscopy would enable them to catch the problem before it became apparent with the PET-CT scan.

And that's exactly what happened.

The one to be taken by surprise is the cancer

Less than four months had passed after ending chemotherapy, when one of the markers, the CEA, began to take a slow but constant path upwards: at each exam the values were higher than at the previous one although only slightly. The PET-CT scan taken only 15 days earlier, the first test which was done at three months, had been negative, but Helen and Leonard were worried, they feared that in one place or another, the cancer was reappearing. They immediately arranged to have a gastroscopy done, even though Helen had had one little over a month earlier. The specialist noticed a small lesion, a little button on the mucosa. "I might not have ever noticed and I probably wouldn't have considered it particularly important - he honestly said – if I hadn't known the case history".

The pathologist found cancer cells in the biopsy, a confirmation that they were dealing with a recurrence of the cancer in the stomach, caught right at its birth. When examining biopsies, pathologists don't usually describe with great detail everything that they see: they limit themselves to say that they see cancer cells, if they are many or only a few, if they have formed a mass or not, and they describe some features of the cells. Leonard wanted to know what was happening in that little button, where the cancer was starting up again so he personally went to study the slide at the microscope together with his pathologist relative. He was amazed by what he saw.

The cancerous cells were immersed in an abundant mucous full of CEA, the marker that had been slowly increasing in the blood. They were sparse and isolated, and seemed to be swimming in that sea of mucous and CEA. Attached to some of the cancer cells, there were CD8, immune system cells that are able to bind to ill or foreign cells and kill them with "lethal blows". Here and there, there were neoplastic cells which showed clear signs of suffering, even if many others seemed to be in good health. Strangely, there weren't any blood vessels, strangely, because the little button was around 5 millimeters in diameter, and a tumor of that size needs these vessels. How could all of this be explained?

The microscope was probably showing them a battle field. The cancer cells were having problems because they were under attack by the body's immune defenses and possibly also by the tamoxifen. At the same time though, they were able to resist and grow. The CEA was probably a great help to these cells.

Leonard went to study the CEA and came across fascinating research, which showed that this isn't simply a glycoprotein that, once released by the cancer cells in the proliferation stage, passes into the blood and acts as a marker of tumor growth. It is a molecule which helps the cells survive in difficult circumstances, and resist anoikis, the death that occurs when they remain isolated and loose contact with the other cells and surrounding tissues, when "they are without a home" like the word anoikis literally means. It may have been thanks to the lake of CEA that they were floating in, that the cells of that small button were able to survive, even though they were isolated and even without any blood vessels. So the presence of that much CEA confirmed the fact that the cancer was having difficulty, but was in any case a reason for concern, because the CEA, aside from helping the cells survive in difficult conditions, also helped them to migrate and become implanted in other parts of the body.

From the idea of strengthening the hormone therapy to the discovery of non-aggressive therapies

What to do? There were those that recommended a change in the hormone therapy. In Leonard's opinion though, there weren't valid reasons to think that the tamoxifen was ineffective: it seemed to be working in other parts, and even may have been working against the cells in that little button, which did seem to be having trouble.

Of course, the tamoxifen therapy was insufficient and needed to be reinforced, but to a certain extent it was working. Otherwise, that little button would have become a large mass, it's cells would have multiplied in the stomach and from there the cancer cells would have gone on to colonize other sites, to further metastasize. Cancer does this, we shouldn't delude ourselves! It was important to take advantage of the early detection of the disease's return and gain from being in advance.

Leonard thought that the ideal would be to add a non-aggressive therapy to the tamoxifen, which wouldn't expose Helen to other risks, wouldn't create other problems for her, and would permit to her of continuing to live as well as she was now. In his search for mild treatments, Leonard explores the scientific literature, and finds quite unexpected worlds.

He became interested in metronomic anti-cancer therapy, which in the past few years has been timidly creeping into clinical practice. It is a kind of chemotherapy which is administered continually, at low doses, and preferably by mouth, so it is easy to take at home, like many other pharmacological treatments that people take during their lives. He analyzes it carefully, it's action mechanisms and clinical results, and begins to think that it could be applicable in a case like Helen's, in which we must keep at bay a cancer which is just raising its head back up after having been attacked by a traditional chemotherapy treatment. Metronomic chemotherapy, in fact, more than killing the cancer cells, puts them in a condition in which they have trouble disengaging themselves, growing quickly, and diffusing themselves.

Leonard seriously studies BRMs (biological response modulators), which could raise the immune defense response. He finds very interesting the mushroom extracts that come from traditional oriental medicine, and in a short time, he becomes an expert in the material, a cold and balanced expert, who appreciates the good in these remedies while understanding their limits.

What pushes Leonard to occupy himself with BRMs, is above all the CD8s that he had seen under the microscope. If the tumor site is a battleground, a direct attack on the tumor cells is not the only possible strategy. It's worthwhile to try to boost the organism's immune response. One of the ways in which the metronomic therapy works, is by making the immune defenses more combative against the cancer cells. Mushroom extracts which will reinforce the immune system in other ways can be added to this treatment. Other methods used to stimulate the immune system don't convince him, especially because they can cause other problems. The mushroom extracts, on the other hand, are practically innocuous, and provide positive effects such as protecting the bone marrow and the liver from the damaging effects of chemotherapy.

Reflecting on the Japanese approach

While studying metronomic chemotherapy and BRMs, Leonard finds himself more and more immersed in Japanese scientific literature. He particularly appreciates two principles which he seems to understand about the way that the Japanese think about treating cancer: to avoid being too aggressive thus making the patient feel even worse, and to keep in mind that the cancer is fighting against the organism, and that, in addition to attacking the cancer, treatments can tend to modify advantageously, the cancer-organism balance.

The example of UFT in mammary cancer helps us understand the first of those two principles. After having surgically removed a tumor from the breast, as adjuvant therapy - that is, as a therapy that is given in addition to surgery to help prevent recurrences or metastases -, in the west, heavy regimes of polychemotherapy, an administration of several chemotherapeutic agents given in the vein, are used. The Japanese make extensive use of UFT, a drug which can be taken orally, and is not particularly toxic. Through large and careful clinical studies, they have shown that taking UFT for a few years give similar results to six cycles of CMF, one of the polychemotherapy regimens used in the west, with the difference that the patient can enjoy a much higher quality of life, and avoid many risks.

The second principle (trying to modify the cancer-organism balance) is illustrated by the case of PSK or Polysaccharide-K, an extract of the Coriolus Versicolor mushroom. In Japan it has been being used in cancer treatment for more than 30 years. It is known that it works by stimulating immune defenses, and also by challenging the cancer in other ways. Clinical studies have demonstrated that it increases the effectiveness of chemotherapy, in particular using UFT in the treatment of gastric, colon-rectal, pulmonary, and mammary cancers. For this reason, in Japan PSK is approved as an anti-neoplastic drug.

In the U.S, and in other western countries, it isn't well known. It isn't approved as a pharmaceutical, but is sold as a dietary supplement. The experts are somewhat skeptical, and seem to ignore Japanese scientific literature. Why is this? There are probably many reasons. One of these might be that it is difficult for western medicine to accept a non aggressive treatment, which modifies the cancer-organism balance and works to support other therapies without being decisive on its own. It is believed that to be successful we need to take a single therapeutic action which is effective. We sometimes don't realize that success is multifactorial, and is the product of many factors that happen simultaneously in the organism to make it possible. Any one treatment that we use is only one of the factors at play, and as important as it may be, can never be the only one.

If this is the way things are, why not act in many ways at the same time? Why put all of our trust in only one remedy? Why focus on one single therapy which we believe to be decisive, underestimating the advantages of combining it with other treatments which could be helpful?

Could it be because of the collectivist culture and the tradition of ethnomedicine?

Helen and Leonard are social science scholars: in addition to psychology, they are quite familiar with sociology and cultural anthropology. When Leonard tells Helen the story of UFT and PSK, they both think about two aspects of Japanese culture that might be able to explain the less aggressive treatments and the focus on cancer-organism balance.

The Japanese, like other oriental peoples are collectivists, differently from westerners who are individualists. For an individualist, one's self is independent from others: to him, what one is, is first and foremost what he thinks and does on his own, autonomously. Collectivists on the other hand have an interdependent self, they feel that what one is, depends on the fact that he is part of a specific social group, and the relationships that he has within this group. The individualist can easily think that he is capable of living on his own, the collectivist only sees himself existing as a part of the group which he belongs to.

If we recommend to a western woman, who has been operated on for breast cancer, an adjuvant therapy with CMF, she will almost certainly accept, even when we explain to her that the treatment will last for several months and that it will be necessary for her to go to the hospital for the venous infusions of the drug. The benefit that she can gain seems to highly outweigh any discomfort or inconvenience that it may cause.

A woman from a collectivist culture is much more likely to refuse or at least, seem perplexed. Going to the hospital for months makes her feel uprooted, cut out of her social group, with the result that her self is compromised, she is no longer herself. At the end of the day, an adjuvant therapy can only reduce the risk that the cancer will metastasize, not eradicate the disease. In the eyes of a woman from a collectivist culture, this benefit seems modest compared to the harm of being partially uprooted for a several months. And so it becomes important to find a lighter treatment which can be completed at home orally, and without changing the everyday lifestyle of the patient, a treatment like that using UFT.

The Japanese, like other easterners have a long tradition of ethnomedicine on their shoulders, which is made up mostly of extracts taken from the natural world and whose use is based on practical experience over the millennia. They have developed a scientific medicine which is among the most advanced in the world, but at the same time, haven't forgotten their ethnomedical heritage. They look with respect at some traditional remedies, even if they then subject them to the rigorous scrutiny of scientific research. PSK is one of the many mushroom extracts used in ethnomedicine that merits our attention because in different scientific studies it proved itself to be effective.

The most important part of the heritage of ethnomedicine isn't in the traditional remedies that science has recycled. It instead lies in the method, the approach, the thought processes that goes into the treatment. Ethnomedicine doesn't begin with the idea of eliminating the cause of the illness: the bacteria, the parasites or the cancer cells. It tries to reestablish a balance which has been broken, so that the individual can be well even if he continues to have the illness and even if the bacteria, parasites, or cancer cells remain inside of him. This is why traditional treatments tend to be less aggressive and emphasize the principle that being well is the important thing, not winning a battle against enemies to our health.

This time the remote opinion is disappointing

Leonard wants to reinforce the hormone therapy by adding to the tamoxifen which Helen is already taking, both UFT and PSK. His idea is to use UFT in a metronomic manner, that is, continually and in low doses. The PSK should be able to contribute by making the immune system more combative. Together with the UFT he intends to administer calcium levofolinate or LV, a vitamin which increases its action, not only because it's a standard combination, but also because it seems that LV could help against possible resistances caused by the CEA. This strategy convinces him essentially for two reasons: it plays ahead of the game and it uses light weapons.

Even though he is already convinced, Leonard decides to get a remote second opinion from the specialized center that he consulted at the time of the diagnosis and that had helped him arrive at the conclusion that the cancer came from the breast. Comparisons are always useful, and all that needed to be done was to write a clinical report, insert it into the website, and wait a few days for the response.

It was the same doctor as last year who gave her opinion, and she was in agreement with the mammary origin. This time though, the doctor rejected Leonard's idea to reinforce the hormone therapy adding UFT and PSK to the tamoxifen. In her opinion it was best to stick with the standard procedure methods, whereas Leonard wanted to change methods. In the standard approach, modifying the therapy is justified only if it is clear that the illness is advancing.

One marker, the CEA has increased, and a residual of the cancer cells in the stomach has been sighted, that little button which worried Leonard, but these aren't strong enough reasons -according to the report- to cause us to act, because they don't authorize us to say that the illness is progressing. According to the criteria of the UICC (Union Against Cancer), there is progression only when there are clear clinical symptoms, such as growth or diffusion of the tumor which is visible using a PET scan, or radiological examinations.

This opinion encourages them to repeat the PET scan in a few months and to change the treatment only if clear signs of progression of the illness are shown. If the situation isn't particularly bad, it would be sufficient just to replace the tamoxifen with a different hormonal drug, otherwise she would need a new chemotherapy. It's the"wait and see"approach, as it is habitually called by many oncologists, the rule of being patient, monitoring the situation and intervening only if things get worse.

Leonard has the exact opposite in mind. He wants to anticipate the game Having found the illness returning in a part of the body when it's comeback is at the very beginning, is to him an advantage which shouldn't be thrown away. Precisely the fact that for now there is only one small button in the stomach, permits them to more easily block the illness, and gives them a higher chance for success. To wait would mean to find ourselves having to deal with a more serious illness, which would be harder to manage.

Formalisms

Leonard is disappointed by the opinion, also because some of the things written are debatable, and leave him perplexed. To say that we need to remain inactive, just because the criteria decided upon by an organization such as the UICC say that there is no progression seems absurd to him. It means giving excessive importance to conventions, to protocols, to general recommendations that experts give, while losing sight of reality.

The illness is returning to the stomach: gastroscopies and biopsies have helped us to discover it. The UICC criteria are based on radiological signs because we are usually able to discover progressions when they become visible with these exams. Helen's case though, is different, a case in which thanks to the gastroscopy, we were lucky enough to notice the comeback of the illness earlier, before it started showing radiological signs.

In the report, the doctor wrote that the analysis of the biopsy shouldn't be taken into consideration when making therapeutic decisions. She finds interesting the considerations about the CD8, which make us think about a battleground, and the CEA which could help increase the survival of the cancer cells in a hostile environment, but in practice thinks they should be ignored. In the end, we have to apply the rule which says that we should only consider histological exams which are routinely used in order to orient the treatment plans. Once again, Leonard asks himself until what point we should follow the rules. If we have useful information which could help us to better understand the case that we're treating, and to further tailor the treatment, why not use it? We should definitely use it with caution and wisdom, but it would be a pity to throw it away.

Scientific inaccuracies

It is written in the specialist's report that UFT doesn't give good results with mammary cancer. But Leonard knows a lot about the vast Japanese experience, in which this drug is used after operating on this type of cancer. He has read with much interest articles on the subject, which have been published over the last few years.

The doctor later tells him, that if anything, he could use capecitabine instead of UFT because they are very similar. Leonard knows though, that UFT and capecitabine differ from each other in multiple ways, one of which he finds very important. The side effects that capecitabine causes, can make it difficult to continue giving capecitabine for more than a year. The Japanese on the other hand, habitually use UFT for two years, and in colon cancer, for three. He'd read about cases in which patients had taken UFT for five years, and at times even more than ten, without major problems. Leonard hopes to be able to treat Helen's illness for a long time, and he likes the idea of using a drug which can be used long term.

The report also contains an affirmation which Leonard finds disconcerting. Hormone therapy drugs like tamoxifen, and chemotherapy drugs like UFT - in the doctors opinion - shouldn't be used together, because they can interact negatively with each other, one can reduce the effectiveness of the other. This idea circulates among oncologists, it is based on a few reports, but it doesn't have a real base. In Japanese clinical experience, tamoxifen and UFT have been used together and have given good results, even better than when used separately. Studies show that they actually are synergistic, which means that they strengthen each other. Chemo-endocrine therapy, the association of hormonal and chemo therapies, is in fact practiced and is interesting, but many oncologists harbor prejudices against it. They make negative judgments about it based only on hearsay, because it's fashionable to discredit chemo-endocrine therapy, without going to read up on it seriously.

In subsequent years, the ideas of oncologists have changed, albeit slowly. In any case, at the time that Leonard was making his decision, prejudices against chemo-endocrine therapy were the norm, and the saying "don't mix hormone therapy, with chemotherapy" was common. Fashions which come and go.

Faulty reasoning

The doctor who wrote the opinion asserts that the tamoxifen was probably not working any more. We can already say this with assurance, even if we'll only have the final proof that it isn't working on the day when we see progression according to UICC criteria. At that point, we'll change from tamoxifen to a different treatment.

This line of reasoning doesn't make sense to Leonard. It contradicts itself by saying that the tamoxifen isn't working anymore, while at the same time stating that we should behave as if it were still working. However, in Leonard's opinion the biggest error in this way of thinking, is that it begins with the idea that the tamoxifen is either working or not working, without leaving any middle ground.

The illness was originally diffused over the whole stomach, the peritoneum, the ovaries, and the ureter. Cancer cells are definitely still present in all of these sites, seeing as how chemotherapy even in the best of cases always leaves a small percentage of cells which it isn't able to kill. In any case the illness was now returning only in a small area of the stomach. Why is this? It's reasonable to think that in other areas, the tamoxifen is keeping the cancer cells in line, or at the least, slowing down their regrowth.

Furthermore, in the part of the stomach where the cancer is coming back, it's growing quite slowly. The biopsy also suggests that the cancer cells are encountering some difficulties. It could be that to some extent, the tamoxifen is working even there. So why discontinue a treatment that could be at least partially working? For as long as possible if there aren't problems, it is better to go ahead adding new treatments to the old ones, instead of substituting them.

In the report, there is a scientific observation which is mostly correct: we don't have proof that UFT is effective against metastatic mammary cancer which has previously been treated with other methods. There is some truth in this, seeing as how the Japanese use UFT as an adjuvant, to help block recurrences and metastasis after a mammary cancer has been surgically removed. So in this Japanese experience UFT is the first chemotherapy that woman with breast cancer are treated with, and it is used when there isn't metastasis.

Even taking this into account, the doctor's way of thinking still doesn't make sense. It starts with the idea that there isn't enough evidence that UFT works with a metastatic breast cancer which has already been treated with other methods, and ends saying it doesn't work, and therefore shouldn't be used. But without sufficient study, we aren't actually able to say whether it works or not. The lack of proof that it works doesn't prove the opposite. To be sure that it doesn't work we would need wide experimentations in which the UFT didn't work in metastatic breast cancer. We don't have any such proof.

In any case, to Leonard's way of thinking, there are other more important things to consider. Seeing as how there is a complete remission and the PET scan is negative, Helen's situation is similar to that of a woman whose breast cancer has been removed, and who is now trying an adjuvant therapy.

Even more important, is his decision to use the UFT in a metronomic manner, which means using it continually, and with low dosages. Differently from traditional chemotherapies, metronomic chemotherapy has an effectiveness which doesn't depend very much on the type of cancer. And thinking about it, metronomic UFT has been experimented with quite successfully in different kinds of treated metastatic cancers, including breast cancer. It should be repeated that all that Leonard wants is that the UFT together with the tamoxifen and the PSK, help to keep Helen's illness at bay.

Leonard does what he thinks is right,
and the little button disappears

Leonard is disappointed by the remote opinion, but still finds it useful. The objections stimulate him to think, to dig deeper, to study and to think about his thinking, to reason about the reasonings. Because of this hard work, he now has clear in mind the reasons for his decision to add UFT/LV and PSK to the tamoxifen. He annotates them in thirteen points, which he writes in a short paper of a few pages.

Stephen T., the oncologist who had suspected mammary cancer originally, and had recommended the chemotherapy which had worked so well, reads the thirteen points and says that he is in agreement with Leonard. While reading, he lets a little laugh escape every now and then, like someone who discovers that ideas which he believed in have their limits, he laughs seeing how our human presumption crumbles in the face of reality. In the end, he summarizes his thoughts like this: Leonard's choice isn't standard, but it makes the most sense. He goes even further: if treating cancer only entailed following protocols, it would be better to send all of the oncologists home, and be treated by computers.

Helen asks Leonard to illustrate all of his thoughts in detail. She reads the thirteen points, and is present when Stephen T. says that he agrees with Leonard. At the end of the day the last word is hers, "I agree, lets add UFT/LV and PSK to the tamoxifen". Her reasons are simple and clear, "It is unacceptable for us to wait and not do anything while the cancer is already returning to my stomach, and I like the idea of not taking things too far, and of going ahead adding one non-aggressive type of therapy to another non-aggressive therapy".

Helen immediately begins taking UFT with levofolinate, but nearly a month passes before they have PSK to add to the treatment. Leonard had studied the production techniques of the mushroom extract, and doesn't trust supplements which are for sale in the west, he prefers to use the original Japanese drug. So he orders it from a pharmacy in Tokyo.

The CEA gets lower, and after five months, nothing more can be seen in the stomach. The physician who performs the gastroscopy seems surprised, and in order to be sure, takes biopsies in the area where the little button had been found. The biopsies are negative, there are no more cancer cells. Once again we have a complete remission.

The luck of having discovered how to overcome diarrhea

In five months the illness has regressed, but it hadn't been easy. After the first few weeks of UFT therapy Helen had diarrhea with several stool losses per day, which stops only after taking multiple loperamide pills, a drug normally used in these cases to treat diarrhea. At times Helen is forced to stop taking the UFT and to stop feeding herself, and has to rely for days on intravenous administration of liquids and nutritional substances. Luckily Leonard is there, and he is able to do all of the treatments in their own home.

The effects of the diarrhea make Helen feel bad, so much so that she is weak and fatigued even if she walks up a slight climb. We can't continue this way, with so much suffering. The UFT therapy was supposed to be non-aggressive, but it is proving to be unsustainable.

Diarrhea is a typical side effect of UFT, a drug which also provokes intestinal inflammation. The association with levofolinate can also increase the risk of diarrhea. Leonard has read some scientific articles which were written by Japanese authors with much experience with UFT, which said that diarrhea can be dealt with without causing major problems. But how?

Leonard suspects that there must be expedients, diarrhea management strategies that the authors take for granted and don't mention in the articles. So he starts to consult Japanese scientific literature, in a desperate research for useful information. He discovers fascinating ways to deal with the problem.

Aim at the cancer cells mostly during the night

One expedient for avoiding diarrhea is to chronomodulate the UFT administration, this means to appropriately distribute the drug over the 24 hours of the day. The highest dose is usually given in the morning. This is a mistake, because this way even with the same effectiveness, we see many more side effects, including the intestinal damage which causes diarrhea. In order to try to reduce the damage, the highest doses should be given between midnight and two in the morning, so that the drug reaches it's highest blood concentrations in the middle of the night.

UFT, like most chemotherapy drugs, attacks cells while they are reproducing, it blocks and damages them while they are dividing and multiplying. It is able to kill cancer cells precisely because they are in reproductive phase. But the cells of the intestinal mucosa also multiply themselves, they do this because the mucosa renews itself, and must replace cells which die and are eliminated. For this reason the UFT also ends up damaging the intestinal mucosa, which in turn, causes inflammation which provokes diarrhea.

At night, the cells of the intestinal mucosa rest, and their reproduction activity slows down. Cancer cells on the other hand, continue replicating according to their own rhythm, and are unaffected by the time of day or night. This is why giving the highest dosages during the nighttime is better. During the night, the high doses of UFT mainly attack the cancer cells which continue with their replication, while sparing the intestinal cells which are at rest.

With the drug fluorouracil, chronomodulation is frequently used: when it is administered by intravenous continuous infusion, the largest amount of the drug is given at around four o'clock in the morning. Strangely though, chronomodulation isn't commonly used with UFT. Even though UFT is a prodrug of fluorouracil, which means that it is converted into fluorouracil and works through this drug.

Melatonin, taken before going to sleep can help to reinforce the chronomodulation. It is the substance in our body which regulates our sleep rhythms, and which is taken regularly as a supplement to treat both insomnia and jet lag, a condition that comes after long airplane trips where multiple time zones are crossed. It tends to block the replication of healthy cells during the night, including those of the intestinal mucosa, and keep them, in a certain sense, as if they were sleeping, whereas it isn't able to slow down the replication of cancer cells. So if a patient takes melatonin, the UFT treatment affects the intestinal cells even less over the night.

In addition, melatonin isn't toxic, and seems to cause a series of other favorable effects, for instance it strengthens the tamoxifen treatment, stimulates the immune system, and seems to make the chemotherapy drugs more effective while reducing their toxicity, and possibly causing other difficulties for the cancer cells. It has been used without causing major problems at least for short periods of time with dosages of 30-40 mg per night. Leonard thinks that in Helen's case 10-15 mg a night might work well.

Let the organism rest over the weekend

UFT is usually taken for three or four weeks, followed by a week's break. In the beginning Leonard follows the standard procedure and Helen takes UFT for three weeks followed by a week of rest. While exploring scientific research, Leonard finds Japanese research that experiments with a weekday-on/ weekend-off schedule, where the drug is taken from Monday to Friday, and Saturday and Sunday are rest days. The articles that he finds state that a weekday-on/ weekend-off schedule is just as effective, if not more so, than the standard one.

Leonard thinks that this weekly schedule, apart from being effective, should also be less toxic and might be able to resolve their problem with diarrhea. The harm that the drug can cause to the intestine and to the body in five days is definitely a lot less that the harm it could cause in twenty one or twenty eight days. And so in theory the treatment should give us less problems if we give the body a weekly rest, even if it's for a shorter time. While continuing with his studies, Leonard finds subsequent research that confirms his theory: the weekday-on/ weekend-off schedule is in fact much more easily tolerated by patients.

Google Translate gives him a hand this time. The most recent articles, those of the research that demonstrate the better tolerability of the weekly schedule, are in Japanese. Leonard and Helen, with much patience, translate them with the help of the Internet.

Protect the intestine

Supplements and pharmaceuticals can protect the intestinal mucosa from the damage that UFT causes. The glutamine which Helen had been taking earlier to combat the cachexia could help. Several clinical studies clearly show that it reduces the harm to the intestinal mucosa caused by chemotherapy. There have been some studies which show that it can be helpful to treat diarrhea, but other studies don't confirm this. For this reason, guidelines in the United States don't recommend it to treat chemotherapy induced diarrhea, whereas in Canadian guidelines it is among the treatments recommended.

Leonard's impression is that it would be foolish not to give Helen glutamine. The simple fact that it could help to keep the mucosa healthy is enough of a justification, moreover it is harmless, and according to some studies could even help to fight the cancer. The fact that it isn't always able to reduce the diarrhea by itself doesn't mean much, only that it should be used together with other treatments. Sometimes the authors who write the guidelines think in quite a strange way.

In Japan zinc carnosine, is a drug which is approved particularly for gastric ulcer. In the West it is sold as a dietary supplement, and is used to treat stomachache and gastritis. Studies using animals suggest that zinc carnosine protects the intestinal mucosa from damage caused by chemotherapy and by other drugs which also harm the mucosa. There are few clinical studies using people, and those which exist are done using few patients and are usually for drugs which are different from chemotherapeutics. For Leonard though, the information which we have about zinc carnosine is enough to make him believe that it could be useful to help Helen deal with the UFT treatment.

Zinc carnosine is practically harmless. Some have expressed concern over the toxic effects of zinc which is found in the molecule, so much so that the FDA (Food and Drug Administration), the governmental body in the united states which is in charge of regulating the use of pharmaceuticals and food products, limited its permitted dosages to half of what is commonly used in Japan. This concern though, is unfounded.

It's true that zinc in high doses can cause harmful effects. Among other things it lowers immune defenses, which in Helen's case would be detrimental seeing as how this defense is needed to fight the tumor. But these harmful effects only start when the patient takes more than 100 mg of zinc a day. With the doses of zinc carnosine which are normally used in Japan, there is a daily intake of 34 mg of zinc, around one third of the quantity that shouldn't be surpassed. For this reason, there is no risk. Actually, at this daily dosage zinc can help the immune response and not harm or weaken it.

In Helen's case, zinc carnosine also seems useful for some other reasons. Through a series of mechanisms it reduces the inflammation in the stomach, and helps to create a less favorable terrain for the cancer, which has been starting up again precisely in that area. According to the results of some research, zinc carnosine may also increase the UFT's action against the tumor in the stomach, especially if the two drugs are given together, or at a short distance from one to the other.

Leonard also discovers something surprising. Drugs which stimulate bile secretion and accelerate intestinal transit, that that shorten the time it takes for food to travel through the digestive tract have proved to be useful for managing diarrhea. In the beginning Leonard is puzzled because a quicker intestinal transit rate is usually associated with diarrhea and these drugs could cause diarrhea. Should we treat diarrhea with diarrhea? After reflecting on it though, he finds that it makes sense. If the intestinal content moves more rapidly, the UFT remains in contact with each intestinal segment for less time and does less harm. The intestine is a tube which is several meters long. If the UFT crosses it more quickly, it distributes it's damage over a very large surface and the damage becomes minimal at any specific point.

A whole year of ceasefire

Leonard believes it is appropriate to use all of the remedies which, according to his studies might be useful to treat the diarrhea: chronomodulation, a weekday-on/ weekend-off schedule, and drugs and supplements which could help protect the intestine. He shows them to Helen, explaining to her with great detail how they work. To illustrate some of the complex mechanisms he uses intricate models with arrows, plus and minus signs, and abbreviations such as IL-6, IL-8, IL-10, NFkB, HSP27, HSP72, ROS, MMPs, etc.

Helen doesn't get discouraged, she asks questions, and question after question leads Leonard to help her understand more or less how things stand. At the end she decides: what are we waiting for?

Thanks to the expedients that Leonard discovered, the diarrhea miraculously disappears. The UFT therapy becomes doable. Leonard doesn't know if their success is due to one or more of the expedients used, or if all of them worked together to remove the diarrhea. Thinking about it though, he doesn't care: what matters is that Helen is taking the UFT, and feels good. Helen is happy even though she has always liked going to bed early and sleeping peacefully, and so taking pills between midnight and two in the morning is hard for her, especially in the beginning.

Eliminating the diarrhea has allowed Helen to take UFT, the UFT works, and the cancer in the stomach regresses. It is a time of ceasefire again. Their fight against cancer has stopped, but only for the moment. Helen and Leonard are both aware that sooner or later it will be back.

The ceasefire lasts a year. Helen and Leonard take advantage of their time to study and write articles and books about psychology, sociology, and cultural anthropology. These are their subjects, subjects which they have dedicated themselves to for decades and which they love. They also continue with organizational consulting for businesses, teach students, and hold training courses for adults. They work a lot, it's as if they're trying to do as much as possible while they still can.

During a ceasefire it's important to observe the enemy. Every fifteen days they have an appointment for the cancer markers, every two months for the gastroscopy, and every three months the PET appointment. At each appointment Leonard feels a sense of anxiety, a strong sense of anxiety which doesn't go away until he gets the results back from the tests, results which give them hope that the ceasefire will continue. Helen, as usual, seems calmer, colder. She justifies her coldness saying that sooner or later every one of us will die, that we know this since childhood. When Leonard goes too far with his anxiety she threatens him: if you keep on behaving like this, I won't take care of myself any more.

More aggressive than before, the disease reappears in the stomach

This time, Leonard is more concerned than usual when he goes to the gastroscopy appointment, because over the last two months a tumor marker, the CA72-4, has slowly but constantly been rising. Leonard has noticed that the levels of chromogranin and gastrin in her blood have also been increasing. This leads him to believe that the environment in her stomach has been changing and becoming more favorable for cancer cells.

The gastroscopy shows something astounding, a large plate of inflamed and thickened mucosa, where five neoplastic nodules can be found, five masses of cancer cells. The situation is unbelievable because only two months before there hadn't been anything there, the stomach had -at least apparently- been normal.

The specialist says only "I'm sorry". Helen and Leonard read a sense of surrender on his face, possibly an idea that the game has become serious again, that there is no more way to be able to deal with the situation with non-aggressive therapies, to continue to live well.

The biopsies are positive, there are cancer cells both in the nodules and in the thickened inflamed mucosa around the nodules. Leonard hurries to have Helen do a PET scan, which confirms the illness's presence in the stomach. The year of ceasefire is over.

An incredible remote second opinion

This time Leonard doesn't think to ask for a remote opinion from the specialized center that they had consulted in the past: he already knows that they will tell him that it's time to go back to chemotherapy, and that maybe he was mistaken in not following the standard approach. He tries contacting another well known center which also gives remote opinions about cancer. Their response is even more disappointing. The doctor that writes back doesn't give them any advice about the treatment, but disagrees with the diagnosis: he thinks that the cancer originates in the stomach and not in the breast. He concludes saying that the doctor who is treating Helen doesn't seem to be expert enough, and that he would be willing to take over her care.

Leonard and Helen are disconcerted and bothered, by the rude attempt at stealing a client, and even more so for the ignorance that he demonstrated.

This oncologist bases his treatments on his own practice, he blindly believes in his own opinions based on practical experience, and without a crumb of humility, happily ignores the scientific research and thought processes that lead us to believe that the cancer comes from the breast. He doesn't even ask himself why this gastric cancer responded so well to treatment (unfortunately, stomach cancer doesn't usually respond well to chemotherapy) especially with a treatment that usually works better in breast cancer than in stomach cancer.

Here we have a type of doctor that is sometimes seen, and is best to stay as far away as possible from.

Two possibilities that Leonard and Helen reject: returning to chemotherapy and removing the stomach

After the squalid chapter of this remote second opinion, Leonard and Helen go back to Stephen T. he is an important reference point for them. He is the oncologist who had intuited the mammary origin of the cancer in the first place, and had recommended the chemotherapy which had proved a winner. The next year he had agreed with Leonard and given up the protocols which had been so important to the doctor of the remote opinion, and had gone along with the idea, which had also proved a winner, of strengthening the hormonal therapy that had nipped in the bud the disease recurrence in the stomach.

Stephen T. sees two viable possibilities: repeating the chemotherapy, or going with surgery and removing the stomach. The strategy of strengthening the hormonal therapy by adding non-aggressive therapies has blocked the illness and let us gain a year. Now though, the cancer is back in the stomach in a serious form. The non-aggressive therapies are clearly not enough anymore.

Everything leads us to believe that the cancer will get out of control if we don't use more aggressive and decisive treatments.

With everything considered, Stephen T. prefers the option of chemotherapy, possibly still using docetaxel, which had worked so well in the beginning. He thinks though, that it would be worthwhile to hear a surgeon's opinion, and evaluate the other possibility, because at the moment the illness seems to only be present in the stomach. The idea of removing that part of the body and possibly being free of it is tempting.

Leonard is hesitant and isn't afraid to tell his reasons. He finds it unjustified to use chemotherapy which he considers an excessive weapon when the cancer is confined to one site only, a specific area of the stomach. In Leonard's opinion using chemotherapy makes sense when the illness has spread through multiple parts of the body, like it had been in the beginning of Helen's illness. With this treatment in fact, we are able to treat the illness in almost the whole body. But it doesn't make sense to shoot everywhere, if our goal is to reach only one specific spot. Too many side effects to bear! Helen might suffer from the treatment without a good reason. The option of chemotherapy doesn't convince him, also because it doesn't give them any guaranties of success. The probability that it will work is slightly under 50 %, less than in one case out of two. Another reason to consider it an extreme remedy, to be used only when we don't have any other options and it seems like all is lost.

He has two reasons to be against the hypothesis of surgery: quality of life is greatly reduced without the stomach, and the idea of completely freeing ourselves from the cancer is an illusion. A gastrectomy whether total (the removal of the whole stomach) or partial (the removal of only a portion) causes problems (a sense of fatigue, feeding problems, nausea, bloating, pain, etc) and it normally takes a few months to get back to a somewhat normal life.

Undergoing such suffering would make sense if we could be certain, or at least have a good probability that we could get rid of the cancer, but we are in fact quite sure of the opposite. In the beginning, the illness had been spread outside of the stomach, in the peritoneum, the ovaries and the bones. Some cancer cells had definitely remained in these sites, it is as if they are only resting and are inactive. Among other things, the stress of surgery could reactivate them. If that should happen, we would have resurrected an inactive illness in the hope of getting rid of it.

At this point, Stephen T. has a lot of respect for Leonard. He has begun to think that there is something really special in the way that he's trying to take care of Helen's cancer. So he listens with interest, and at the end says, "It all makes sense, but how do you think that you'll be able to keep the illness under control without using chemotherapy or surgery?".

Leonard believes that it is appropriate to continue with the same treatment, but change it somewhat to make it work better. He illustrates the two things that he thinks should be changed: modify the gastric environment to make it less hospitable for the cancer, and treat the illness locally, but without removing the stomach, either partially or completely. He already has some ideas, however he needs to study more to come up with a precise strategy.

Stephen T. remains silent for a few minutes as if taken by surprise by the change of perspective which Leonard suggests. He says, "I agree, let's try, but let's give ourselves a deadline, a few months, no more".

Simple moves to modify the gastric environment and seeing the first results

Helen has been taking lansoprazole, a pump inhibitor that a gastroenterologist had prescribed to her at the beginning of her illness. Pump inhibitors are drugs which are commonly used to treat gastroduodenal ulcers and other conditions, and are frequently given to patients with stomach tumors. In general, a less acidic gastric environment can be useful when there is a tumor, mostly because the mucosa is less prone to inflammation. However, pump inhibitors can have effects which could possibly make the gastric environment more favorable for cancer growth. When Leonard puts all the scientific information available on the subject together, he immediately realizes that giving Helen lansoprazole had been with great probability a mistake.

Pump inhibitors alter the secretion of a mucous which protects the gastric mucosa, they compromise gastric motility, and most importantly, inhibit somatostatin production. This hormone, secreted by delta cells in the stomach reduces the presence of molecules which can help cancer growth (gastrin, cholecystokinin, IGF-1), molecules which are also produced by other cells in the stomach. Somatostatin, in addition, through other pathways contrasts inflammation and helps keep acidity under control. Patients who take pump inhibitors have less somatostatin in their stomachs, and for the cancer cells this is an advantage.

Leonard decides to substitute the lansoprazole with ranitidine, an old drug which reduces acidity without lowering the somatostatin, and which doesn't cause the problems of pump inhibitors. He adds octreotide to the ranitidine. The octreotide is a somatostatin analog, which means that it has the same effects as somatostatin while being a different molecule.

Research seems to show that somatostatin analogs demonstrate a series of effects that work against cancer, even if trials have given disappointing results, apart from particular cases for short periods of time. But Leonard only wants to modify the gastric environment, he isn't interested in using octreotide as an anti cancer drug. It doesn't bother him that in theory octreotide could have anti cancer activity, such as tending to block angiogenesis, the job of creating new vessels which the cancer uses for it's growth, or regulating immune system activity, but he doesn't delude himself.

Stephen T. understands Leonard's intentions, partially because he's an expert of somatostatin and octreotide. Other oncologists though, refuse to understand that Leonard is only trying to create a better stomach environment which makes it harder for the cancer to grow and spread. They believe that cancer can be fought only with methods that attack it directly.

The results are somewhat surprising. At the gastroscopy a month later, only three of the five original nodules are present. The plate of thickened inflamed mucosa has disappeared: the three remaining nodules are now inside an apparently normal mucosa. The CA 72-4, the marker which had increased, drops back down again. Chromogranin and gastrin return to normal, which is a sign that the gastric environment has improved, as Leonard had hoped it would. The result is surprising, because it is based on two very simple changes, based on thoughts about the biochemistry of the gastric environment: substituting lansoprazole with ranitidine and adding octreotide.

Helen isn't very happy about her new treatments, because octreotide is given three times a day with injections under the skin in the abdomen. She has always hated injections, and the idea of having them in the belly is new to her. She closes her eyes and mouth when Leonard gives her the shots, visibly, as if to create a barrier and separate herself from them. But in any case, she is happy with the results that it gives, and finds them worth the three shots that she has to take every day, or even more if necessary.

EMR and PDT do the rest and the stomach goes back to being clean

The two simple moves to modify the gastric environment have given good results, but they are clearly not enough. The illness in the stomach is still there, even if it has improved. Leonard is also well aware that cancer cells are good at adapting themselves to hostile conditions. For this reason, when we make the environment less hospitable for their growth, we have to expect that after a first moment when they find themselves in difficulty, the cancer will start growing again, in the same way or even more than before. That's why the other action that Leonard has in mind is essential: treating the illness locally, being able to destroy the tumor in one way or another, without removing the stomach.

Fortunately it is easy to get inside the stomach with endoscopy. But how can we clean out the stomach? Which endoscopic treatments should we use? Leonard goes to study the possible endoscopic treatments, and after thinking long and hard, goes with an EMR PDT combination.

EMR (Endoscopic Mucosal Resection) or mucosectomy is a surgical technique which allows us to remove nodules which are present on the mucosa of the digestive tract, such as those that Helen has in her stomach. It is a surgical technique, but a minimally invasive one, it causes as little damage as possible, because it is delicate and precise. It is done by entering the stomach with an endoscope, a pipe with a video-camera attached which is used for the exam, the nodule is taken by a snare, which when pulled, cleanly cuts off the nodule at it's base and cauterises the wound.

PDT (Photodynamic Therapy), is an ingenious way to destroy cancer cells. It was invented in the beginning of the nineteenth century, but has been greatly developed since then. A photosensitive drug, a drug which has a particular reaction to light, is injected intravenously. This drug spreads throughout the body and is also absorbed by the tumor. At this point the area where the tumor is gets lit up by a light at a specific wavelength. The photosensitive drug in the tumor is activated and causes an oxidative stress which damages the cancer cells, both directly and indirectly through it's effects on blood vessels and on the immune system.

It's worthwhile to combine the two treatments. The EMR would by itself remove the nodules. But the rest of the cancer cells in the surrounding area would still be there. Furthermore these cells would end up invading the ulcer caused by EMR and prosper there. PTD can remove the rest of the cancer cells and guaranty a good result.

Where can they go to treat the cancer in Helen's stomach with a combination of EMR and PDT? Leonard has trouble finding a suitable center. EMR is done nearly everywhere, but there are only a few centers in the world where they do photodynamic therapy in the digestive tract. Among other things, even when used, it is normally done in the esophagus, and not in the stomach. Luckily, Leonard has an important font of information: scientific literature, where he can see which centers publish clinical experience with PDT, and he can also check the results that they obtained.

In the end, Leonard finds a center which seems good to him, not only because it is famous, but mostly because Edward B. operates there and manages the department. He is a researcher who has much experience in the field, he has developed many innovations, and seems to be open minded.

Scientific papers usually include the e-mail addresses of the authors. Leonard finds Edward B.'s address in one of his publications and writes to him, he tells him about the case, and asks if he would do the combined EMR PDT treatment for Helen. Edward B. writes back immediately and accepts: in his opinion, Leonard's idea is a good one, and is worth trying.

The center that Leonard chooses is far from where they live and they will need to take a long trip in an airplane. Helen and Leonard haven't done much traveling in their lives, especially not by plane. They deal with the experience with interest and with a bit of satisfaction, as if the illness has given them a gift, the gift of novelty, which mitigates all the anxiety and uncertainty of the treatment.

They set to work to organize the trip, finding a comfortable hotel on the internet, and booking it. The clinic is welcoming and different from what Helen and Leonard are used to. Treatments are done on an outpatient basis, and there is no need to stay in the hospital. So they can look about and act like tourists in the preparation days leading up to the procedure. Above all, they notice how organized the big famous clinic is, they look and study, like they are used to doing whenever they see a new piece of the world.

The treatment works. After a month the gastroscopy shows that her stomach is back to normal, there aren't any signs left from the illness which had seemed to be so aggressive and difficult to treat.

Now the choice of avoiding chemotherapy and the stomach removal surgery seems to have been guessed. Helen and Leonard are satisfied, Leonard breaths a sigh of relief: he had thought of an unusual and courageous strategy against Stephen T.'s advice, and it had, at least for the moment, worked.

An encouraging misunderstanding

When Helen makes an appointment for her EMR PDT treatment something happens that Helen and Leonard find funny and which reassures them. It pushes them to go faithfully ahead along their chosen path. In that clinic the first thing that new patients have to do in order to make an appointment is to send a report from the doctor who is treating the case to the appointment center, which then sends the request to the specialized department. So after talking to Edward B., Leonard prepares a detailed clinical report, that Helen sends to the appointment center.

Unexpectedly, they get a response from the oncology department, not from that of gastroenterology where Edward B. works and where Helen is supposed to go to for her treatment. The oncologists discourage them from taking the trip to be treated there, seeing as how Helen is being very well cared for by the doctor who is treating her where she lives. "We - writes the oncologist who signs the response - couldn't do any better".

What had happened? By mistake Leonard's report had been sent to the oncologists instead of to the gastroenterologists. The oncologists that had read the report had then mistakenly thought that Helen wanted to go there to treat her cancer in oncology, and not only for EMR and PDT in the gastroenterology department.

It may have been the clinical report that Leonard had written which had caused the confusion. It had been very detailed, and told the story of Helen's cancer from the beginning, with all of the clinical reasoning, doubts and the audaciousness and successful decisions. Leonard ends the report recommending a local treatment with EMR and PDT, and requesting to have the treatment done there. Evidently though, the doctors who had read the report had been so attracted by the body of the report and had focused on that and missed the point at the end, the request which was meant for them.

Nothing more than a misunderstanding, quickly resolved when Leonard told Edward B. what had happened. Helen and Leonard in any case find this misunderstanding important. Without meaning to they have asked for a remote second opinion form a prestigious cancer treatment center, and the response had been "we couldn't do any better".

The price of photodynamic therapy

During the procedure everything goes well. Helen undergoes the infusion of Photofrin, the photodinamic drug, in a welcoming hospital room, assisted by a diligent nurse and with Leonard at her side. After the phleboclysis they go back to the hotel, and two days later she undergoes the EMR and PDT therapy. In reality, she notices almost nothing because she is sedated and it feels to her like having an hour of deep sleep. It is Leonard who lives the moment with worry and commitment, both before and after the treatment he talks with Edward B. and discusses the clinical decisions.

After a day though Helen begins to feel poorly: she has stomach pains, nausea, and vomits if she just tries to take a drink. Leonard tries to help her with medicines for vomiting and pain. In order to prevent dehydration, Leonard gives her intravenous liquids. When the day that they have to leave comes Helen is feeling much better and can manage the airplane journey.

The biggest discomfort is caused by problems with light. After a photodinamic therapy, one must avoid light exposure for at least a month if not more. The photosensitive drug remains in the body for a long time. If skin and eyes are exposed to the sun or other light sources for a few minutes, they could become inflamed or burned. Because of this after photodinamic therapy one must stay out of the sun and take precautions.

Helen and Leonard are very organized. They've bought high altitude sunglasses on the internet which have a high level of protection from the sun. They found elegant gloves and a stupendous wide-brimmed hat in a boutique, which together with a silk shawl would perfectly cover her face. For the rest of the outfit, she wears long trousers and a long sleeved blouse. Dressed in this fashion Helen has something intriguing about her, and in her way, is fascinating. She knows this, and behaves accordingly, she enjoys playing this part when the occasion arises.

After the treatment, Helen and Leonard plan to meet their sons and daughters in law in Rome, the eternal city, for a short holiday. It's September and certain angles are very beautiful. Helen and Leonard walk around with their sons and daughters in law, enjoying restaurants, museums and monuments. At times, it seemed that Helen's clothing choice is nothing more than a touch of elegance. The illness is now forgotten.

Living like this though, is tiring. They must always be on their guard: distractions can't be tolerated, uncovering herself, even if by mistake, could be dangerous. They also must keep the curtains closed to prevent the sun from coming in and always make sure wherever they go that the lights are LED and not traditional light bulbs.

The disease reappears and Leonard understands that a change of paradigm is needed

The stomach is back to normal, thanks to the combined treatment with EMR and PDT. The PET scan has gone back to being negative, and the cancer markers are fine. After a few months though, when they go to do a routine gastroscopy, they find a nodule, a small tumoral mass right in the area which had just been treated.

When Leonard sends an update via e-mail to Edward B., he responds disappointedly, "I was hoping that the treatment would work better". Seeing as to how there is only one nodule, and it is a small one at that, Helen and Leonard decide to have it removed with EMR in a clinic closer to home. They go without the PDT in order to avoid the long trip. They agree to go without it also because such a short time has passed since the last treatment. The Photofrin, the photodynamic drug is eliminated slowly by the body. So when the treatment is repeated after such a short time, the drug accumulates in the body and thus the risks of light exposure increase and there are more problems to manage.

The results are nevertheless disappointing, Helen and Leonard regret having been so lazy and optimistic. EMR normally leaves a scar which needs time to heal. In Helen's case, the scar has been invaded by cancer cells and has become a neoplastic ulcer. This is not a nice outcome, because neoplastic ulcers tend not to heal, and they can dig deep, penetrating the stomach wall. A failure, but a useful failure which helps Leonard get to the core of the problem.

Evidently it is mistaken to think that we can eliminate once and for all the disease in the stomach, to eradicate it. The right thing to do is to continue to treat it periodically. We need to go with the idea that tumor cells are present in the stomach mucosa and that new lesions will continue to sprout. We mustn't delude ourselves about this. The important thing isn't eliminating the disease once and for all, but continuing systematically to treat the disease each time that it starts to sprout.

All well considered, the final result is the same. If we systematically remove each new lesion which starts to grow, the illness will almost certainly not progress, it won't expand in the stomach, and it won't spread elsewhere. Helen will be doing as well as if we eradicated the disease. Isn't this what we want? The only real difference is that if we aren't able to completely remove the cancer, Helen will have to continue to go through treatments. But this is a reasonable price to pay, if we use easily tolerated treatments, that don't cause to much difficulty to her daily life.

Leonard has discovered a new way of thinking about local treatments, a new paradigm. He understands how different this idea is from the traditional paradigm by reflecting on the words that Edward B. wrote him, "I was hoping that the treatment would work better". Why should we be so disappointed? If we think about it, the treatment had worked well. For a few months everything had been silent. The point is to accept the idea that no therapy is forever. After reflecting, it seems to him that Edward B.'s words are tied to the sense of frustration that a person who is committed to doing a good job and is disappointed by the results might feel: words that express a psychological disappointment, more than the fruit of a cold and objective clinical evaluation.

Cryotherapy: a resource for withstanding through time

Photodynamic therapy isn't suitable for what Leonard has in mind, mostly because it can't be safely repeated with the rhythm that one wants. Photofrin, if repeatedly injected at regular intervals tends to accumulate, and so the body becomes increasingly sensitive to light. Other drugs which are metabolized more quickly can be used, but they seem to be less effective, and are difficult to find. There is also this fundamental fact to take into consideration: Photodinamic therapy has caused Helen much suffering and discomfort, if repeated regularly, these treatments risk ruining her quality of life.

Leonard goes about searching for the right therapy, which can be done safely on her stomach, and which can be repeated regularly without problems. He is leaning towards cryotherapy, which is also called cryosurgery or cryoablation. It's a way to destroy cancer cells that goes back to the 1800s, even further back than photodinamic therapy. The English doctor James Arnott tried to use cold temperatures to treat breast, uterine, and skin cancers using salt and chopped ice. After the second half of the twentieth century more and more advanced technologies were developed to treat prostate, esophagus, liver, skin and breast cancers, and other illnesses.

In the esophagus cryotherapy is done by inserting a tube in endoscopy and then spraying liquid nitrogen on the tumor which is frozen at around -200° Celsius. Cryotherapy isn't commonly used for stomach tumors, but freezing a stomach tumor is easier and safer than freezing one in the esophagus. So there is no reason not to try cryotherapy in Helen's case.

There is also no reason to believe that by some strange chance it shouldn't work. Freezing at such low temperatures should at first dry the cancer cells out and then causes them to burst. After a few hours the arteries that bring blood to the tumor will close, and the lack of blood ends up damaging the neoplastic cells even more. Some well known facts make it appealing: freezing leaves the tissue scaffold intact, the repairs are rapid and well done, and there might be a vaccination effect, because the debris of the neoplastic cells stimulate the immune system.

What convinces Leonard, is the fact that cryoablations are usually well tolerated. They don't cause serious problems in the esophagus and at the most cause slight side effects, so we can expect that in the stomach it should be even safer and cause even less problematic disturbances if any at all.

The game of metronomic therapy and cryotherapy

Thinking about Helen's treatment and putting together various scientific knowledge, Leonard becomes more and more convinced that repeated cryoablations are what is needed. Helen continues with her metronomic therapy with UFT. At a certain point, Leonard realizes that combining the metronomic therapy with the repeated treatments could be a winning move.

The cancer cells present in the stomach can be found in three different stages. Many cells are isolated and dormant or form small masses of a millimeter or less. These cells should be kept at bay by the metronomic therapy, and grow very slowly. In fact, the

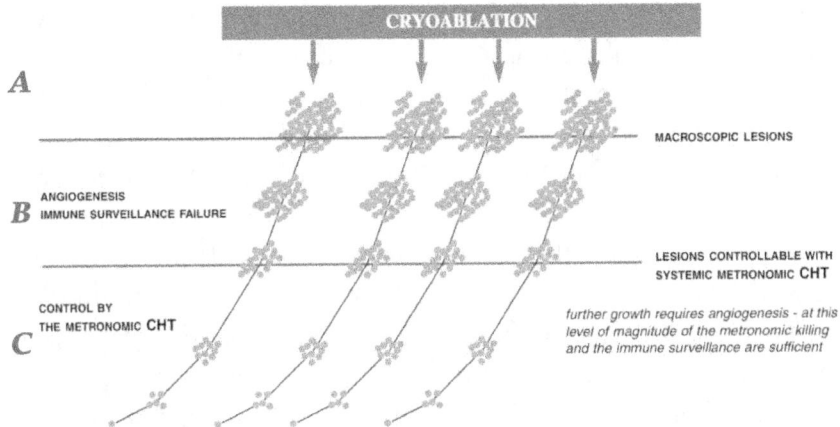

Leonard's model of combining metronomic therapy with cryotherapy

At the C level there are the cells which are kept under control with the metronomic therapy. At the B level, we find cells which have gotten out of control of the metronomic therapy, they are growing rapidly, but haven't yet formed visible masses. Those which have already formed visible masses are represented in the A level. When cryotherapy is done, these are the cells which are seen and treated.

metronomic therapy works through mechanisms (angiogenesis blockage, that is, the blockage of new blood vessel formation, and strengthening of immunosurveillance, that is, the immune system's job of patrol and protection) which work as long as the cells are isolated, dormant, grouped together in small nuclei.

The cancer cells have gotten out of control of the metronomic therapy when they start to form masses of more than one or two millimeters. At that point, they are able to produce the vessels that they need, and to avoid the immune system's action. They replicate much faster in this phase and faster and faster: the growth which was slow, becomes exponential. It's as if they unhooked themselves from the organism's defense control, and from the treatment. But it isn't necessarily true that they can be seen clearly with a gastroscopy, or with a PET scan. They will only become visible when they form large enough masses.

This is why the combination of metronomic treatments and cryotherapy is so useful. As long as the cells are kept under control by the metronomic therapy, this is what takes care of the situation. When they get out of control, and form large enough masses, the repeated cryotherapy intervenes to destroy them. In the midst there is a layer of cells which will remain undisturbed. But it is precisely because they grow so quickly that these cells can be quickly found and destroyed. It would be absurd to put all of our trust in metronomic therapy, and on the other hand it would also be absurd to give up on repeated local treatments. That would give the cancer a free pass.

Leonard builds a model that graphically represents his thought process about the combination therapy. Helen, who is good at computers, and with graphics, helps him transform his model into an elegant graphic, made up of images and texts. It isn't a waste of time, because in this way, the two of them find a way to enjoy themselves while fighting the cancer, and because ideas, once put into a graphic, become stronger.

Years of peaceful war

The idea of going ahead with metronomic therapy while at the same time using repeated cryotherapy treatments in the stomach works. Helen has the treatments every two or three months. Some lesions are seen in the stomach each time, but the illness remains stable, and always in the same area. Each time Leonard and Edward B. decide how long to wait until the next treatment. They base the decision on the situation, sometimes anticipating, or postponing the treatment by 15 days or so.

Helen perfectly tolerates the cryotherapy. It doesn't give her any problems, it is as if she isn't doing it. In the twentyfour hours after each treatment, she observes a liquid diet of fruit juice, milk, and ice creams which melt directly in her mouth. Helen does this in order to carefully follow the prescription, and at the end of the day, she is not sorry. Altogether, she feels really well.

Helen and Leonard are at war against cancer, it is always present in the stomach, so much so that it can be seen at each appointment. The war is calm though, and mild. The only hard side is the worry that the illness might all of a sudden, one day, wake up again, become aggressive, and escape our control, possibly moving to other parts of the body. The travel, the administrative details, the treatment procedures, and the diet after the treatments are all things that they get used to and which start to become part of their day to day routine, their normal life.

This is now their life, and it's not that bad. They become regulars at the place where Helen has her treatments done. Doctors, nurses, and administrative employees in the clinic greet Mrs. Bee like an old friend. The same thing happens in the hotel, with the receptionists and cleaning staff, in the restaurant where they know her favorite foods and beverages, and where they know that after her treatments, Helen always has an ice cream. Years pass in this manner, and the cryoablations are counted in the tens.

Leonard clears up the doubts of Edward B. and his colleagues

Edward B. willingly accepted doing repeated cryoablation treatments. As time passes though, he starts to show some perplexity. At one point he asks Leonard "when are you thinking to repeat the chemotherapy?". Then, as if to justify the question, he adds "my colleagues here ask me". Evidently, in the clinic, they have been talking about that strange case of metastatic breast cancer, that has been going along for years by means of repeated cryotherapy, even though the norm is to treat metastatic cancer with chemotherapy.

At the moment, Leonard limits himself to answer that Helen is using a metronomic chemotherapy, and that he doesn't see the need to treat her with traditional chemotherapy, seeing how the illness is confined to that one spot in her stomach which is easily reachable with local treatments. In any case, in their conversations, both in person and through e-mail, Leonard notices that Edward B. continues to have some doubts.

Edward at times goes back to talking about chemotherapy, and above all, sometimes seems worried about the fact that each time, with each cryotherapy treatment, the tumor is still there, present in the stomach, at times a bit bigger, at others a bit smaller. It seems that he has difficulty accepting the idea that the cryotherapy is working, even if it doesn't completely eliminate the tumor, but merely keeps it stable, always there, and more or less the same.

For this reason, Leonard decides to make the rationale of the repetitive treatments explicit. He writes Edward B. an e-mail which clarifies the key points, in an incisive and direct manner.

Dear Edward,

I think that the treatment up to this point has been a great success. Definitely more effective than chemotherapy. We know very well that years ago, when we found the progression in the stomach, the standard chemotherapy had a response probability of 30 -60 %, that means that in 40 to 70 % of cases, it was unsuccessful. In one or two out of three cases the disease would go ahead despite the chemo.

We also know that after the response to an effective chemotherapeutic treatment, the illness will almost certainly progress again within a year. How many chemotherapy treatments would we have done at this point? Would they have worked? How would my wife have been feeling for all this time? As well as she has been and still is today?

I'm convinced that the strategy of repeated cryoablations and continuing with a mild metronomic chemotherapy, aiming to keep the disease in line, is a winning strategy. Even though, in theory, we can think of eliminating the disease from the stomach once and for all, it seems more reasonable to give ourselves the more modest goal of avoiding local progressions which are difficult to treat, and reduce the likelihood of repetitions in other areas of the body.

The goals of treating metastatic cancer are, prolonging the patient's life and giving them a good quality of life. We are meeting both of these goals. Of course, if we could see the illness disappear once and for all from the stomach, we would be happy, and celebrate a victory. However, if this doesn't happen, if the illness stays there, but my wife continues to live a normal life, the treatment is perfect. We doctors tend to think of cancer as an acute disease, but in reality it is chronic.

I would be very happy to see my wife continue to undergo a large number of cryoablations in these wonderful conditions. Each time that I come to you with Helen, we wish each other "a hundred of these treatments".

You are doing a great job.

I am forever grateful for the help that you're giving me with treating my wife.

My warmest greetings,

Leonard

This time Edward B. leaves behind all of his doubts about the treatment. He responds to the e-mail with a simple "Thank you Leonard", and from that moment on, he goes ahead cleaning the stomach, with conviction. At the first chance he gets, Leonard shows the model that he made together with Helen to Edward B., who examines it with interest. Maybe even his colleagues have second thoughts, seeing as how Helen's treatment from that moment on has officially been called a research case, a case to study to open up new interesting paths.

After years of peaceful war,
the markers interrupt the routine

Thanks to the repeated cryotherapy treatments, the markers remain normal, and the PET scan is negative: even if the gastroscopy every time shows small lesions to be treated, the PET scan doesn't see anything in the stomach. At a certain point though, two markers, the CEA and the CA 72-4, seem restless: at times their values are high, and then they go back down again. They tend to be above the normal levels, as does the serum HER-2, a marker which at those values usually indicates that metalloproteases are at work. These are enzymes which promote the invasion of surrounding tissues by neoplastic cells.

Leonard is worried, and, convinced as he is that they have to act preemptively, he begins to ask himself what is happening, and what can be done to deal with it. He reflects on the possibility of changing the hormone therapy, because of the simple fact that it has been many years now that Helen has been taking the same drug, tamoxifen, and that resistance to long term hormonal therapy is highly probable.

Leonard consults with Stephen T., who repeats the rule of the standard approach: hormone therapy should be changed only in the presence of a clear progression. Here we only have a certain movement of the markers, and so all that is left to do is wait. Leonard, at first, accepts the recommendation to wait and see without hurrying. However he shows his doubts about the standard approach. When we have certain signals, the ideal would be to try to find out what is going on and intervene early, adjusting the therapy with small moves, without upheavals.

On the other hand, in Helen's case the problem of defining progression is embarrassing: on the one hand we have been in progression for years, since the time when the illness came back in the stomach, on the other hand, we are not in progression, seeing as how the disease is under control in the stomach.

Even though Leonard allows himself to be convinced to wait, he knows quite well that they need to be on their guard, and expect the need to intervene from one moment to the next. The alarm rings, and the years of peaceful war, for now, are over.

Helen and Leonard once again refuse chemotherapy

After around four months, the CEA and CA 72-4 rise. Luckily the PET scan doesn't show presence of the illness in other parts

The raising of the tumor markers

Leonard was accustomed to reporting the data of the markers in a specific graphic. You can immediately see when looking at the graphic the increase of the CA 72-4 and of the CEA. A short time after the beginning of the new hormonal therapy the markers go down.

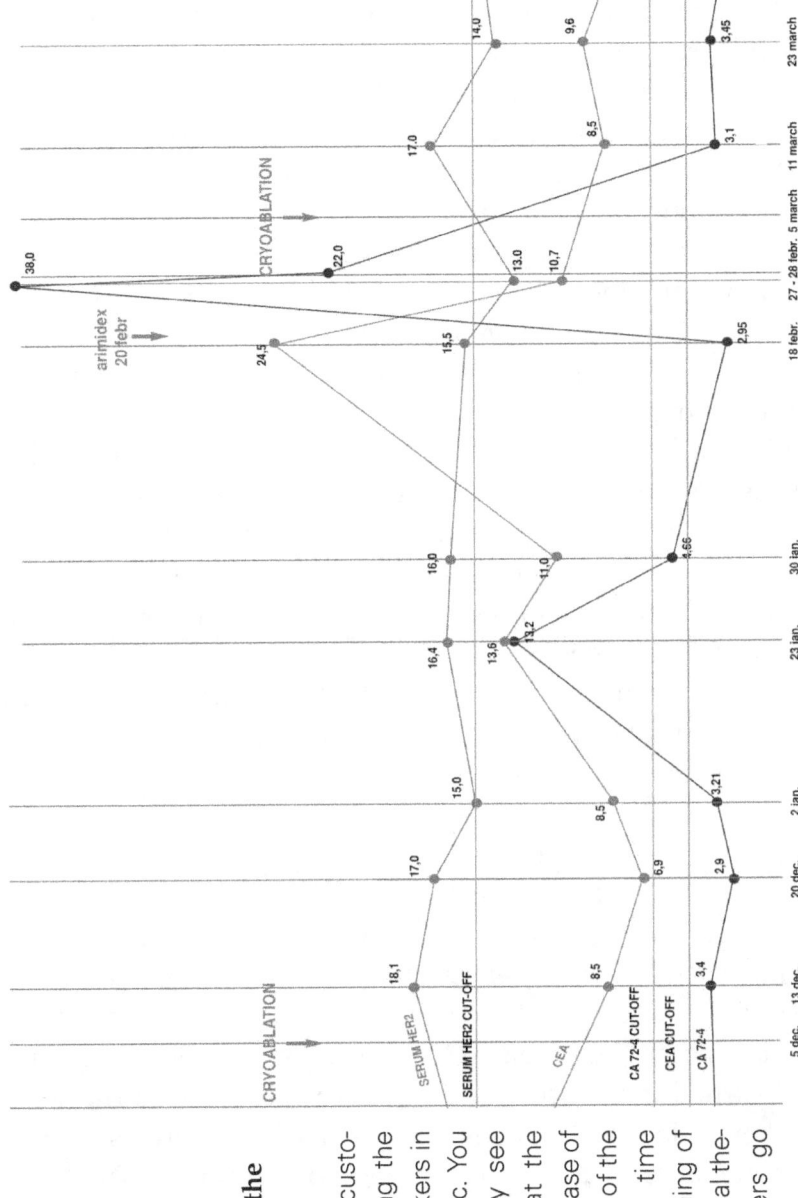

of the body. But in any case this scan shows the disease in the stomach after many years that it hadn't been seen there.

Leonard tells Stephen T., who at the beginning says only that maybe the time has come to act. The next day, he sends Leonard an SMS from the airport where he is leaving to go to a conference "Listen, I don't want to be a pessimist, but I'm under the impression that the illness has become aggressive, I think it's time to go back to chemotherapy. It's been many years now. We should be satisfied. After all, it's a breast cancer and has responded well to docetaxel. Afterward, maybe we can think about changing the hormone therapy".

Helen and Leonard talk about it, and also this time they decide against using chemotherapy. Deep down, what reason is there to use it? The illness is still confined to the stomach, where the periodic cryotherapy keeps everything clean. Helen says, "If you sweep every day, your house stays clean". It's probably true that the cancer has become more aggressive, but that only means that we have to be more careful, and try to think of a way to get it back in the ranks, to try to keep its head down.

The discovery that the stomach produces estrogen

Leonard has many questions that are whizzing around in his head: why is it that the cancer, after the first chemotherapy, reappeared in the stomach? Why is it that it is able to survive in that precise spot in the stomach? What is it that has changed recently that turned the cancer more aggressive, and raised the tumor markers? He starts to study, and just like what always happens with intensive study, question by question, and answer by answer, he learns something that he never would have expected.

There are cells in the gastric mucosa, the parietal cells, which produce estrogen, the female hormone which stimulate breast cancer, and which the hormone therapy tries to counteract. This fact is clearly demonstrated by some Japanese researches, who also found other things which could be interesting in Helen's case. The part of the stomach that produces the most estrogen is the same part of the stomach where Helen's cancer thrives, and is able to survive in spite of the treatments.

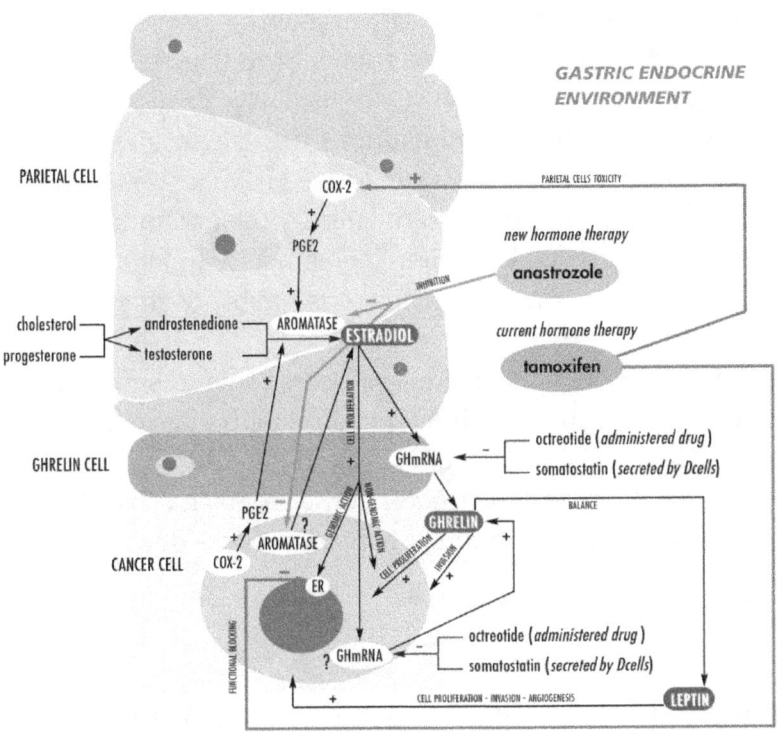

Leonard's model of the gastric environment

The parietal cells of the stomach produce abundant estrogen through aromatase. They do this starting with androgen which they are capable of producing on their own, without needing to use androgen that arrives through the blood. Estrogen stimulates neoplastic cells and favors the production of ghrelin and leptin, which then stimulate the tumor. Inflammation favors this whole process, and tamoxifen can irritate and contribute to setting off this process. Because it is a inhibitor of aromatase, anastrozole might be able to reduce the estrogen in the gastric environment and slow down the tumor growth.

The parietal cells of the stomach produce estrogen via aromatase, an enzyme which converts male hormones into female ones. These cells are also able to create male hormones on their own. The estrogens, with a cascade, can induce the synthesis of other hormones (ghrelin and leptin) which also help the cancer. The quantity of estrogen produced in the stomach is high, and becomes even higher if there is an inflammation.

These facts, along with some others, give Leonard an idea of what might be happening in the stomach. He makes a complicated graphic in order to demonstrate the intricate situation. The estrogen production must have increased in that spot in the stomach. This might have been stimulated by the inflammation caused by the treatments. Tamoxifen has difficulty functioning in an estrogen rich environment, because it isn't able to stop the estrogen from stimulating the cancer cells.

At this point it seems obvious to Leonard what should be the next step to try: substitute the tamoxifen with a aromatase inhibitor, an AI, a different hormonal drug that works by blocking the enzyme which produces estrogen in the stomach cells. There are multiple aromatase inhibitors, Leonard chooses anastrozole, for several reasons.

The new hormone therapy restores the routine

Helen begins to take the new drug and after around twenty days, the markers drop to normal levels. The result is impressive. Stephen T. comments, "Wonderful, I must confess that I was worried". Edward B. finds the information which Leonard discovered in scientific literature about stomach estrogen extraordinary. He says that even though it is all logical, he is amazed by such a brilliant response to such a banal change.

All in all, Leonard is the least surprised of the three. He wasn't sure of his model, but if the situation was really as he believed, the change had to be drastic and quick. He discusses it with

Francis F. a friend of his who is an open-minded doctor with a lot of experience, with whom he frequently confronts. Francis also finds the response obvious. They wonder together about the rule of changing hormone therapy only in the case of progression. They find it a rule which mortifies the intelligence of clinicians: why shouldn't I change treatments if I have evidence that the disease is changing, and I'm able to think of a likely reason for the change? Prudence is understandable, but with this disease sometimes courage is also necessary.

Disturbing compliments

One day, Leonard finds himself, for other reasons, in his pathologist relative's office, the one who had originally guided them to Stephen T. At a certain point, an unexpected confession arrives at his ears, "I have a lot of respect for you". "Why is that?" asks Leonard. At that point his relative pulls out a statistic which he had just received. "Look - he says - the survival times of people with metastatic breast cancer still aren't very long, and with the form that Helen has, where there is visceral involvement, the survival times are even shorter. You are doing an extraordinary job".

After the success with the change of hormone therapy, Stephen T. goes even further, and tells Leonard, "As atypical as your treatment may be, it has been a success. All of the merit is yours".

Leonard isn't very pleased with the compliments. Deep down he feels bothered by them. He struggle to understand what value these statistics might have. All of his work has been aimed at trying to make Helen feel and live well, without giving much relevance to the statistics about metastatic breast cancer. He talks about it with Helen who immediately and intelligently comments, "The treatments are part of our life, and we don't live within the statistics, on the contrary, it is the statistics that mirror our lives".

The compliments also bother Leonard because they tempt him, like a demon. They make him feel as if he is successful, and encourage him to relax, aware of his talent, but there is still a great need to fight, and we are weak in front of the cancer, always.

The compliments tempt him and they make him feel as if he were on his own. They give him a label, that of a genius, who does things which are strange, but well done. If that's how his colleagues see him, how can he discuss things with them? He will have to do everything by himself, venture into Helen's care as the explorer of unexplored lands. Yet he would like to have companions in his adventure, ready to reason and argue with him about things that are at the limits of our knowledge and our possibilities.

To tell the truth though, he isn't entirely alone. Helen is always ready to discuss with him. Edward B. also routinely discusses with him as does Francis F. who sometimes gets carried away by the fascination of the adventure, in addition to some other friends of his who are doctors. Moreover, his pathologist relative, and Stephen T. haven't labeled him forever, and there is still room to debate with them during the adventure of cancer care.

"Come here, you, please let the patient sit quietly"

The compliments are disturbing. It is also a fact though, that there is much to be satisfied with the achieved results: Helen is still alive, and above all she is living magnificently well. It frequently happens that people who know about her illness, especially if they are doctors or other health care workers, stop to look at her, amazed by her appearance, she seems like such a healthy person. Francis F. says that in reality, what she is doing seems like a beauty and anti aging therapy.

One day a funny incident happens in the PET imaging center where they usually go. Leonard goes to the desk to take care of the paperwork, while Helen sits down to wait in the waiting room. A nurse turns to Helen, and with a disapproving tone, says "come here, you, please let the patient sit quietly". Evidently it had seemed to her that Leonard was the sick person, certainly not Helen.

All of a sudden a new alarm,
the tumor might be going deeper

One day towards the end of the summer, Helen has a cryotherapy appointment. The ward is nearly empty: she is one of the few patients there. Edward B. has just returned from a convention abroad, and has had a long trip. He asks Leonard if he thinks they should do a EUS, the echo exam which would allow them to look deeper to analyze the gastric wall and to look around the stomach. He asks because they've already done this exam many times without finding anything particularly important. Leonard believes that when treating cancer, the monitoring should always be done with extreme care, even when it seems like everything is going well. For this reason he says yes.

Edward B. notices to his great surprise that the echo shows a thickening of the muscularis propria, the deep muscle layer of the gastric wall. It could possibly be caused by the tumor which has penetrated deep until reaching that layer. It would be strange, because the tumor markers are at normal levels, and a recent PET scan doesn't shows any problems. However it's a possibility, and what Edward B. saw should be taken seriously. When Leonard returns home he sets about analyzing the problem. He had asked Edward B. to give him the previous EUS images. In his scrupulous studies of them, he sees that the thickening has actually been there for many months already. For some reason it had escaped their notice.

Leonard gets the CDs of the PET scans performed during Helen's disease. The PET scan is normally performed in conjunction with a CT examination, it serves to locate the position of the lesions that the PET scan detects. CT is an imaging method that gives us a good picture of the stomach wall. Analyzing the previous CT images, Leonard discovers that a thickening of the gastric wall was present even before, for a long time, right there where Edward B. has seen it.

All of these clues lead him to believe that the problem isn't being caused by deeper tumor growth. The thickening has been there for a long time. If it was really caused by tumor growth, after all these months the disease would have spread. In fact, the cryotherapy doesn't go deep enough, and the cancer if left there for such a long time, would have grown, and might have moved somewhere else. It's much more likely that the thickening has been caused by an irritation due to the treatments themselves. But we can't be sure.

The hypothesis of surgery resurfaces

Leonard and Edward B. are concerned about the risk that the tumor is pushing deeper, they're attracted by the idea of removing the piece of the stomach where the tumor has been thriving. Edward B. considers the possibility of a full–thickness resection, a minimally invasive surgery that is performed with endoscopy. Leonard thinks that a wedge resection would be more reasonable. This is a slightly more extensive surgery which is done in laparoscopy, and is particularly manageable if done with a robot.

After much thought, Helen and Leonard once again discard the possibility of surgery. It's true that this time they are only talking about removing a little piece of the stomach, and that there shouldn't be any problems afterward. But in any case, a very important issue remains. Cancer cells are almost certainly scattered in the mucosa of the stomach, even though we can't see them. The surgery would leave a scar which these cells would infiltrate easily. Seeing as how the scar would go through the whole width of the stomach, the cancer cells which penetrate it would be able to bring the disease outside, resulting in a spread of the cancer in the abdomen, just like in the beginning of the story. By acting in this way, we risk bringing the tumor out of the stomach, exactly where we don't want the disease to spread. We are the ones to create a pathway for the tumor, through surgery.

Because of this risk, the surgery should be followed by adjuvant chemotherapy, in order to kill the remaining cancer cells and prevent tumor infiltration of the scar. Helen would have to bear the discomforts of chemotherapy and run the risks that this treatment entails. And it isn't a given that the adjuvant chemotherapy would work, that is that it would prevent the diffusion through the gap left by the surgery. Each chemotherapy in fact has a limited likelihood of success. For this reason, chemotherapy is a good weapon, but a weapon of despair, to be used when we have no other means. All things considered, Helen and Leonard aren't yet at the point of desperation, they still believe that it's possible to act with relative calm.

Two new strategies to try to put the situation right: intratumoral chemotherapy and closer cryoablations

With the surgical option discarded, the problem of what the next step should be is still there. We can't exclude the possibility that the tumor is penetrating in depth. Of course they could convince themselves that this isn't the case: Leonard has good reason to believe that Edward B. is mistaken. However, when dealing with cancer, it's usually a good idea to go with the worst possible scenario to avoid illusions and wishful thinking. Helen and Leonard are well aware of this fact.

Leonard has the idea of using injections of chemotherapy drugs within the tumor between one cryoablation and the next. There isn't a lot of experience with intratumoral chemotherapy, but what there is, is interesting. By injecting the chemotherapy drug directly into the tumor, very high concentrations can be achieved in the cancer cells. Even if these high concentrations only persist for a short time, the effect that this peak creates can be extremely important: with such high concentrations of the chemotherapeutic agent, cancer cells sometimes die within a few minutes. Importantly, concentrations can be reached inside the tumor which are able to kill the cancer cells without causing damage on the systemic level.

An Indian research paper peaks Leonard's interest, in the study poor children were treated with intratumoral injections to save on the cost of chemotherapy it later emerged that these children lived better and longer lives than those treated with the more expensive conventional chemotherapy. In Helen's case, injecting the drug directly into the tumor could work by destroying the neoplastic cells which are too deep in the gastric wall to be killed by the cryotherapy. This type of treatment reaches to about 5-6 millimeters in depth. If the tumor has pushed beyond that, there are some cells which the cryotherapy can't reach, and which the drug injected on site may be able to kill.

After considering the various possibilities, Leonard leans toward methotrexate (MTX), a chemotherapeutic agent which has the advantage of not producing lesions in the injection site, it is different in this way from other chemotherapeutic drugs which cause local damage. This is important, because injecting a corrosive drug in the stomach wall, could lead to a perforation of the wall itself.

In addition, methotrexate works well with the treatment that Helen is already taking of UFT and LV (calcium levofolinate, the vitamin which strengthens the UFT's action). If they are taken in the correct sequence, methotrexate and UFT have a synergistic antitumoral effect. Moreover levofolinate counteracts the harmful effects that methotrexate has on the organism when it spreads in the body after acting in the tumor. The important thing is that the drug kills the cancer cells at the injection site, its effects in other areas, cause damage more than anything else.

Leonard finds a way to go even further. He thinks that by injecting other drugs in the tumor, it becomes possible to enhance the action of chemotherapeutic agents, something that is hard to do with the same drugs administered systemically. So he decides to inject a certain amount of dipyridamole and insulin along with the methotrexate. These drugs strengthen the methotrexate's action, but the attempts to use them together using a systemic administration weren't very successful, because we can't achieve the required concentrations of dipyridamole and insulin inside of the tumor. If the injection is done there directly, we can achieve these concentrations, at least for a period of time. Leonard studies the problem seriously and makes several calculations to determine the doses of insulin and dipyridamole to inject into the tumor to increase the chance of the methotrexate working.

Between one cryotherapy treatment and the next, an expert endoscopist who is a friend of Leonard's gives Helen four or five injections in the tumor, with around a week's distance from one to the next. They don't notice great improvements, but it is already a good result that everything remains as it is: if the tumor stops growing, and doesn't push any further, we should already be satisfied.

Helen tolerates the intratumoral injections very well, with no side effects. But undergoing these injections every week is stressful for her. Helen and Leonard go to a clinic that's around 100 km from their house, so they don't have to travel that much. Helen, however, has to undergo a gastroscopy every week. There is also all the preparation work and the multiple drugs that she has to take at scheduled times, in addition to a series of precautions which Leonard suggests to keep the possible side effects of the methotrexate to a minimum.

Leonard searches for an alternative strategy, another way to get to the cells which are lurking deeply, without stressing Helen. At a certain point he starts to think that the most obvious way would be to move the treatments closer in time to each other, do them around once a month instead of once every two or three months. If we don't give the tumor time to grow between the cryoablations, its width at each cryoablation should be smaller. In this way even if we arrive at most to 5-6 millimeters in depth, we should be able to completely destroy them. He talks about it with Edward B., who agrees and thinks that it's a good idea. The only part that bothers him is the frequent travel. But Helen and Leonard accept the idea of intensifying the trips, hoping to resolve things in five or six months of closer treatments.

This time the markers exaggerate

When Helen does the closer cryoablations, with around a month of time between treatments, the two cancer markers which had been rising previously, the CEA and the CA 72-4, begin on a progressive upward slope: at each test these markers are higher. In particular, the CA 72-4 is growing at worrying rates. In the beginning it slowly rises from 2 to 7, but later on, after each cryotherapy appointment, this marker is double what it was at the previous time, until it arrives at values of around 100 which had only been seen in the beginning when the illness had been widespread.

Usually the first thing to think about when the cancer markers start to rise, is that the tumor may be growing, either in the same place or that it's spreading and growing in other areas. As a general rule, it is thought that as the cancer cells grow in number, the tumor mass becomes bigger, and the cancer markers increase. In Helen's case though, it isn't working that way.

Edward B. carefully examines the stomach, and discovers that the tumor isn't growing more than before. Even with the EUS, the echo-endoscopy, we can't say that it's growing deeper, possibly even less, and we don't see the lymph nodes. Leonard hurries to have Helen do a check up to see if the cancer has spread elsewhere, out of the stomach. The PET scan doesn't show anything outside of the stomach, even when repeated several times. Leonard has Helen take a cerebral resonance test because brain metastasis doesn't show up well with the PET scan. This test also comes back negative. It seems that the only thing there is the tumor in the stomach, which is being taken care of by the cryotherapy treatments.

When we have to say thank you to the mistakes

Each time that Edward B. does the cryotherapy treatments, he also performs some biopsies, taking fragments of the tumor to examine. Seeing as how the markers keep on rising, Leonard asks the pathologist to do a series of tests to try to understand if the cancer cells have changed. Unexpectedly, from the pathologists response it seems that the estrogen receptors which had been present since the beginning, and which had pushed them to use the hormonal therapy, aren't there anymore. Leonard reviews the scientific literature on the topic, and concludes that the pathologist's response is not very reliable. In a breast cancer's history, the loss of estrogen receptors is quite rare. When the test results are negative, it's usually because there have been problems or mistakes in the technical procedures.

Leonard asks to repeat the estrogen receptor tests in all of the available samples and this time they are positive: the estrogen receptors are still there, it had been a false negative. Still not satisfied, Leonard wants to also examine the beta receptors not only the alpha, the only one which is usually determined. He asks the pathologist who had performed these special tests at the beginning of Helen's illness to do the complete profile of the receptors.

This request results in some unexpected yet very useful information. A specific type of beta receptor, the beta 1 which had originally been abundant in the cell's nucleus, are now found mostly in the cytoplasm of the neoplastic cells. These receptors, when in the cytoplasm, can cause a resistance to chemotherapy treatments, as well as to the physical treatments such as the cryotherapy which Helen has been repeatedly undergoing. This is very important, so Leonard asks to have the test repeated with a new biopsy sample. The results are still the same.

What to do? Leonard decides to add another drug, fulvestrant, which is capable of blocking and degrading estrogen receptors, including the beta 1 present in the cytoplasm. He hopes in this way that Helen's cancer cells become more responsive to the cryotherapy. After a few months, the beta 1 in the cytoplasm have nearly disappeared.

Helen and Leonard reflect on how sometimes a mistake can be useful, if the circumstances are combined appropriately. If it hadn't been for the erroneous test result which said that the estrogen receptors had disappeared, Leonard would never have discovered the beta 1 receptors in the cytoplasm and would have never taken steps against them. Helen and Leonard are experts in human error and they know that errors don't always bring about negative consequences, frequently they are innocent, and at times even good.

Even if they know this in theory, they still find the experience stimulating. The pathologist who did the test is embarrassed by his mistake, but Leonard reassures him, and thanks him for his help.

The enigma of markers

The cancer markers, especially the CA 72-4, continue to rise, even though the cancer isn't growing in the stomach or spreading elsewhere. How can we explain this marker's growth?

One hypothesis is that the treatments themselves are making the markers rise more and more. Each time that the tumor in the stomach is frozen, many cancer cells are destroyed and leave debris in the bloodstream. Among these debris are the markers that are found with the exams. This crescendo can be explained if you think that it takes around three months to eliminate the debris from the bloodstream. Since only two months pass between one treatment and the next, at each cryotherapy, new debris are added to the old ones still in the bloodstream, and so the markers continue to rise.

It should also be noted that the markers in the debris can be fragmented, broken into multiple pieces. The blood test might count each separate piece as a full molecule of the marker. So it would give values that are higher than they should be. If all of this is true, then the very fact that the closer treatments are working could cause the values to rise.

This hypothesis seems plausible, but Leonard is skeptical for various reasons, starting with the fact that it's a positive hypothesis and we must apply the principle of avoiding wishful thinking. He starts to work on another hypothesis: that the cancer cells are producing the markers in larger quantities. If each cell produces more markers, these will progressively rise in the bloodstream, even if the tumor mass remains about the same, with the same amount of cells. He arrives at the idea that it might be an alteration in the synthesis of glycoproteins, a so called aberrant glycosylation. Glycoproteins are molecules that usually are around the cells, and the markers, CA 72-4 and CEA, are aberrant glycoproteins of cancer cells.

It isn't a good hypothesis, because it would mean that Helen's cancer cells are becoming more aggressive. More precisely, that they are less likely to form masses, and more likely to move and migrate, with the risk of ending up in other body sites. Recently Edward B. has noticed some small superficial lesions not far from the main lesion, as though they are moving along the surface of the gastric mucosa.

The story continues

Which hypothesis is the right one? The most optimistic, or the pessimistic one? Or are they both true? How can we tell if things are going in one way or the other? And above all, what can we do to change things to our advantage? Leonard works on it, he talks with Helen about what he discovers and the story continues. Their search to get to know the cancer inside of Helen, and their quest to manage it goes forward. This cancer has become their companion for ever. When in a good mood, Helen calls it "my brother cancer", as if to say that at this point they have become inseparable. But when she's struggling, she labels her cancer with epithets which aren't very nice, insulting nicknames. Since she would never say rude words, she uses acronyms and abbreviations, which seem polite, even if the meaning is clear.

Things that we can learn from the adventure of Leonard and Helen

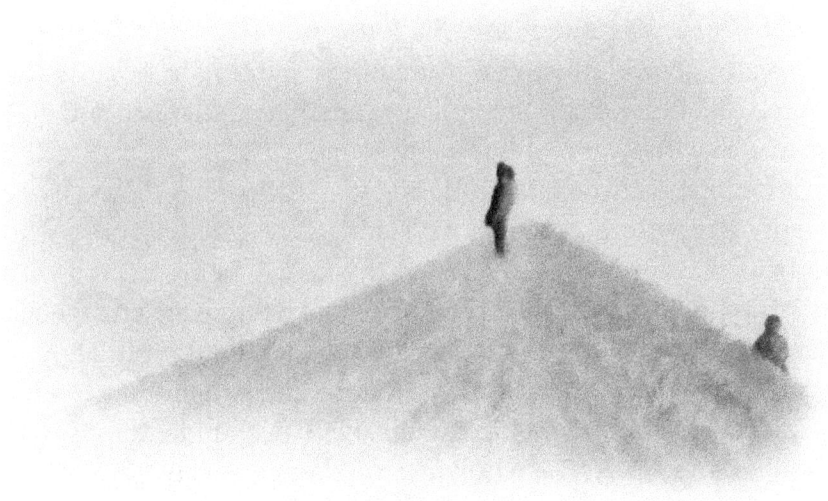

The philosophy of care comes first

Usually, when stricken with cancer, people think that the most important thing to do is to find the right treatment, the therapy which will be capable of saving us from this terrible disease. There are people who, upon discovering the illness, begin to search for the most famous specialists and the best cancer hospitals. Putting ourselves in good hands, and trusting the experts seems to be the most serious way of of finding the right treatment programs, and dealing with the problem.

Others search for less obvious solutions, it is as if they think that in order to deal with exceptional problems, we need to find exceptional responses. There are those that are attracted by miracle cures, unusual remedies that can give unusual responses, hopefully in their specific case. By, for example, going to Cuba to search for scorpion venom, or feeding an intimate hope that a special diet or food supplement can make the difference and give them a chance when traditional therapies fail.

Sometimes cancer patients decide to participate in clinical trials, scientific experiments to test new clinical treatments. Those who participate are usually attracted by the idea of being treated with new methods in a advanced center, where doctors are engaged in cancer research. They don't consider the fact that that treatment, because it's still in an experimental phase, can either be successful, or not successful, and that in "double blind" experiments, it's possible to be among those who are treated with placebo, that is, not treated with anything that works, instead of the real treatment. One must also consider that in order to participate in the trial, the patient has to give up on the use of other treatments, in addition to the fact that cancer research is a very slow process, and so in the best case scenario, only a small advantage can be gained.

Relying on the help of good specialists, and knowing the available therapies is definitely helpful, but the most important thing is the way that we think about treating cancer. We have certain ideas about this illness (what type of disease is cancer? what's the best way to deal with such an illness?), about what to expect from treatments (should we try to be rid of the illness? try to live well? live for a long time? etc), about how to evaluate treatments (when can we consider a treatment as successful? what risks and side effects can be considered acceptable? etc). At every step, we think in one way or another and we make decisions depending on our convictions about these questions. Our philosophy of care, the way we think about treatments, guides us in our decisions. Our success depends, above all, on this.

In Helen and Leonard's story, it's evident that their philosophy of care is decisive. Leonard studies a lot, he reads about possible treatments, and searches for specialists able to do what is necessary. But above all, the success in Helen's care is tied to Leonard and Helen's thought process which leads them to certain types of important decisions: whether to wait, whether to repeat the chemo, whether to add UFT to the TAM, and so on. Guiding their decision process each time, is the way that they think of cancer and cancer care. They're also open minded in the way that people who know what they want and reflect on things usually are. So if their long thought out reasoning leads to a different conclusion, they don't do what certain experts tell them to, or what is normally done.

EVEN DOCTORS TEND TO PUT TOO MUCH STOCK IN THE RIGHT TREATMENTS

Oncologists, as a rule, don't let themselves be pulled in by miracle cures, and they generally are well aware of what it means to participate in a trial. None the less, they tend to think that the important thing is guessing the right treatment. They know from scientific literature the probability that a specific therapy has of working in a specified type of case: for example in non-small cell lung cancer, at an advanced stage, with gemcitabine, we can expect a 20-25% response rate, with vinorelbine, the response oscillates between 15-30%, and with an association of cisplatin and vinorelbine, up to

♦♦♦

30%. With these statistics in mind, oncologists evaluate each case and play their card, hoping to win the round.

Research, at least clinical research, where researchers test treatments, has a similar logic. Researchers work to discover new and better remedies, and decide which one is best depending on the situation. In a certain sense, they work in order to show oncologists the best cards to play in their games.

Because of the fact that doctors concentrate on the problem of finding the best treatment, they tend to overlook the philosophy of care. They don't always give enough importance to the ideas and thoughts about illness and treatments which are frequently crucial for successfully managing cancer.

Why is it that doctors usually concentrate on guessing the treatment, to the point of disregarding ways of thinking that can be so useful in cancer management? Maybe one reason is that looking for the right treatment seems like the most simple and obvious thing to do. Another reason might be found in medicine's history. The biggest successes in medicine have been cures of certain diseases, thanks to the discovery of new drugs that made previously untreatable diseases, treatable all of a sudden. The most spectacular example is that of bacterial infectious diseases. In the past, many people were dying from infections that today seem trivial to us. It was the discovery of antibiotics that changed everything. Deep down, doctors and researchers think that a similar cure can be found for cancer, and they think of it as though it were an infectious disease that we still haven't found the right antibiotic for. But fighting cancer is a difficult test of our times, and can't be dealt with easily, nor by deluding ourselves with medicine's successes of the past.

Cancer is a chronic illness

In order to manage cancer in the best possible way, an idea that we should keep printed in our minds is the fact that cancer is a chronic illness. Leonard says this very clearly in his email to Edward B., "We doctors tend to think of cancer as an acute disease, but in reality it is chronic".

Acute diseases are temporary, they come and go. They frequently go because they are healed spontaneously, or with the help of treatments. In these cases, the illness is only a parenthesis in the person's life. Other times though, the acute illness marks the last moments of life: it comes, and in a short time is gone because we die as a result of this disease. Differently from acute illnesses, chronic ones come and don't go: once they arrive, they accompany us for the rest of our lives. We are able, thanks to the treatments, to manage them in one way or another, and live in better or worse conditions despite the illness, and to overcome complications and risks of death. But the illness is always there with us.

The fact that cancer is a chronic illness is most definitely true in the case of metastatic cancers, those cancers that have spread from the original site and have given repetitions in other parts of the body. If we are confronted with a metastatic cancer, it will be with us for the rest of our lives, whether we survive for a longer or shorter time, and if, in the end, we die from cancer or something entirely different. In any case it is important to realize that in some sense, we are dealing with a chronic illness even when the disease is discovered early, before it gets the chance to spread, when it's still in its original site. We will have to make do with the risk of metastasis for the rest of our lives.

Even though cancer is a chronic illness, there is a widespread tendency to think, and behave as if it were acute. Patients and family members do this, as do doctors, who frequently act as though they had an acute illness in front of them, one that can be wiped out by the right moves, and that in any case is destined to end.

If you think about it, you can understand why we tend to make the mistake of considering cancer as an acute disease. The idea that such a serious disease, capable of killing from one moment to the next lasts forever throws patients, as well as their family members and doctors into crisis. Thinking about it as if it where acute, not having clear awareness of the fact that it's a chronic disease, helps us delude ourselves to believe or pretend to believe, that sooner or later it will be gone. In addition, we aren't accustomed to thinking about chronic illness, because traditional medicine focuses on acute illnesses, with which it has achieved its best results.

As sociologists have shown, in our society when one gets sick, a particular condition is created, a condition which is difficult to bear for long, especially if we think that it will last for ever. A sick person, especially when the disease is severe, tends to be exempted from his commitments and pushed away from the chores of daily life. He has to trust those that are treating him, and has much less freedom and autonomy than before. Others see him differently, and in small ways they treat him like a citizen of another world, and in several ways try to rally around him. Living as a sick person, for the patient himself, as well as those around him, is easier to bear if we think of the illness as acute.

In any case, considering cancer as an acute illness is a mistake, which usually brings with it a series of bad choices. For example, if we consider the illness to be acute, we accept the use of more aggressive treatments, which uselessly attempt to eliminate it once and for all. At the same time, we underestimate useful treatments just because they are not aggressive and don't give us hope of eradicating the disease. We feel beaten, because the illness is always there, when we should be going ahead to fight with a clear mind. Or, on the other hand, we delude ourselves of being free of the illness, just because the cancer, for the moment, isn't showing signs of its presence.

IS CANCER THAT HASN'T GIVEN METASTASIS CHRONIC AS WELL?

In a certain sense yes, Normally a primitive cancer, found before it has spread and still localized in its site of origin, is surgically removed. Thanks to treatment a high enough number of patients are cured and surgeons are usually proud of the outcome. But as hard as they might work on the treatments, there is always a certain probability that, at any moment, the illness will come back, maybe even worse than before. This risk will be with us for the rest of our life.

Take for example, colon cancer. Five years after surgery, 40-50% of patients treated only with surgery don't have a relapse of the il-

♦♦♦

lness. If we add adjuvant chemotherapy, in an attempt to kill off remaining cells after the surgery, the percentage after 5 years of patients who don't have a relapse of the illness rises to around 60-80%. This means that even if we add adjuvant therapies to the surgery, we have a one in three, or one in four chance of having a relapse within five years, either a local relapse, or seeing metastasis at a distance. In later years, the probability of a relapse progressively drops, but it never reaches zero.

There is always some risk. In the best case hypothesis, the illness stays with us like a threatening presence. In fact, this presence is biological. Even in patients who have had the operation, and live the rest of their lives without relapse, there are still probably some cancer cells, it is just that they aren't able to bring back the disease in that time span.

The important thing is keeping in control of the illness, not eliminating it

If we accept the idea that cancer is chronic, the treatment goals become clear: we don't need to try to eliminate the disease once and for all, it is sufficient that we keep it under control, keep it calm, and see to it that it lets us live for as long as possible, while giving us as few problems as possible.

Leonard understands what the real goal of cancer cares should be when he intuits that the time has come to change paradigm. Edward B.'s first treatment, the one with mucosectomy and photodinamic therapy, had been a success, but after a few months, a new nodule was found in the stomach. Edward B. was disappointed, but Leonard convinces himself that they need to go with the idea of treating the lesions each time that they appear, and continue with that method. So he searches for a type of treatment program that doesn't make life difficult for Helen, and that can be repeated over and over. He orients himself towards cryotherapy. He has passed from the paradigm of curing the disease, to one of keeping in control of it.

Leonard clearly explains the paradigm of keeping cancer under control, in his e-mail to Edward B.

I'm convinced that the strategy of repeated cryoablations and continuing with a mild metronomic chemotherapy, aiming to keep the disease in line, is a winning strategy. Even though, in theory, we can think of eliminating the disease from the stomach once and for all, it seems more reasonable to give ourselves the more modest goal of avoiding local progressions which are difficult to treat, and reduce the likelihood of repetitions in other areas of the body.

The goals of treating metastatic cancer are, prolonging the patient's life and giving them a good quality of life. We are meeting both of these goals. Of course, if we could see the illness disappear once and for all from the stomach, we would be happy, and celebrate a victory. However, if this doesn't happen, if the illness stays there, but my wife continues to live a normal life, the treatment is perfect.

If you think about it, why should it be so important to eliminate the illness at all costs? Why aren't you happy just keeping it under control? Imagine that we could be capable of keeping the illness perfectly, or at least almost perfectly, under control. The illness is always with us, but it doesn't bother us, at least not in a serious way. In the end, we die of other causes just like everyone else. What flaws can you find in this kind of care?

It can be helpful to reflect on certain, non aggressive, cancer types, that are only discovered at autopsies. This is the case for example with occult thyroid carcinoma. Frequently, people who have this disease live their whole lives without realizing that they have cancer. Studies have been conducted in multiple countries in the world to see if people who died from other causes, had a thyroid carcinoma at their autopsy. In certain studies, there weren't many people with thyroid tumors that they hadn't noticed, but in other studies, there were many such cases. In one Japanese study, a thyroid carcinoma was present in nearly 30% of autopsies, in a Finnish one they found more than 35%.

Cases like that of occult thyroid carcinoma, plant seeds of doubt about how medicine has approached cancer care. The focus has been about how to kill cancer cells, or how to remove them from the body. Less work has been done to understand what tools we can use to keep the cancer cells under control for the rest of the persons life, like what happens with occult thyroid carcinoma.

Why the habitual use of chemotherapy is mistaken

Usually women with metastatic breast cancer do around one chemotherapy treatment each year, with an average of a treatment every 10-11 months. They live for an average of two and a half years, and spend 30-50% of their time doing chemotherapy treatments. In the many years of her illness, Helen has only done 1 chemotherapy treatment. Her story is different from that of many others because Leonard and Helen have refused the habitual use of chemotherapy. They refused it when the illness reappeared in the stomach, and the doctor from the remote opinion recommended that they wait and eventually go back to chemotherapy. It also happened when the illness came back more aggressively in than before, and it was Stephen T. who recommended the chemotherapy. Then once again, years later when not even Stephen T. held out with that strange treatment without chemotherapy, and said that it might be time to go back to standard treatment.

Leonard and Helen made a good move, if you take a closer look, the habitual use of chemotherapy is mistaken. Why is this? When treating metastatic cancer, an initial chemotherapy treatment is normally done. If there is a response, if the disease regresses, we wait, and do another chemotherapy treatment when it returns. If, on the other hand, the first chemotherapy is unsuccessful, another one is usually attempted as soon as the patient is able to bear it. This is the way that it's done, going from one chemotherapy to the next. Oncologists call them successive lines: the first line, the second, the third, and if possible, subsequent lines. Protocols indicate

which drugs to use in each line, and how to treat heavily pretreated patients, those who have already done many chemotherapy
treatments.

One problem with habitual chemotherapy use is that each time,
the probability of success becomes lower. The cancer cells which survive the chemotherapy, those from which the cancer returns, tend to
be resistant and more capable of surviving, despite the next treatment. They become more resistant precisely because of the chemotherapy treatment that they've undergone. The capacity to endure
attacks, and to adapt themselves to adverse and even extreme conditions, this is a surprising characteristic of cancer cells. So once the
path of chemotherapy is taken, we are condemned to, slowly slowly,
have less weapons at our disposal, and less of a chance to be successful. At the end of the road, with a heavily pretreated patient, oncologists find themselves in great difficulty, they will sometimes try
anything, like gamblers, or if not, they give up.

Habitual chemotherapy use is mistaken also because it ends up
ruining the patient's quality of life. Thanks to the fact that she had the
chance to manage the illness successfully without the use of chemotherapy, Helen lived well for many years, like a normal person. She
worked and lived her life, and in the eyes of others, health care workers included, seemed to be in perfect health. She very much enjoyed when the nurse in the PET scan center had thought that the
cancer patient was her husband, and said to her, "Come here, you,
please let the patient sit quietly". Those who spend 30-50% of their
time in chemotherapy certainly have a much worse quality of life.

There's also another fact: chemotherapy kills. Each time that we
do a chemotherapy treatment, in addition to the risk that it might
not work, there is also the risk that the chemo itself that can cause
death through complications. The likelihood of dieing from chemotherapy varies by the regime, namely by the drugs used and the chemotherapy scheme. On average it isn't high (usually under 1%), but
there still is a certain level of risk, especially going ahead with the
successive lines, or if the patient has heart or liver problems or other
medical conditions. These could be previous problems that the pa-

tient had before the cancer, but they could also be connected with the cancer, or caused be the treatments themselves.

It would be a mistake to jump to extreme conclusions and believe in the idea that chemotherapy should always be avoided. Chemotherapy is a fundamental resource in the fight against cancer. Helen managed to live well, and for many years, thanks to the fact that the chemotherapy that they had done in the beginning, worked, up to the point of giving a complete remission. The point is that chemotherapy should only be used when it seems that the disease isn't controllable with other methods. In a certain sense, chemotherapy is an extreme weapon, that should only be used when the war in the trenches has failed.

The most intelligent strategy would be to avoid chemo for as long as possible, as long as we are able to keep the disease at bay without it. So after each treatment it would make sense trying to put off the next chemotherapy as long as possible, using all possible and imaginable means. This is what Leonard and Helen do.

A large part of Leonard's study is devoted to finding ways to fight the illness without the use of chemo: metronomic therapy and BRMs in addition to the hormonal therapy, locoregional treatments in the stomach, the change of hormone therapy which was suggested by reflections about changes in the gastric environment. Leonard and Helen consider all of the time that they aren't using chemotherapy to be time gained to live their lives, and the longer it lasts, the better it is.

THE LESSON OF ETHNOMEDICINE

Thinking about ethnomedicine helped Leonard and Helen realize that the habitual use of chemotherapy isn't a good idea. Leonard thought that using PSK, a mushroom extract which is approved as an antineoplastic medicine in Japan could be helpful. From there, they started to reflect on ethnomedicine, traditional medicines which are still used in many places in the world, especially in some parts of Africa and Asia, where many people don't have the eco-

▶▶▶

nomic means to buy the products of modern scientific medicine, and where people prefer more traditional treatments.

Ethnomedicine uses extracts taken from nature, mostly from plants, instead of drugs produced in a laboratory. These are called ethnodrugs, obtained with specific extraction procedures. Some modern drugs, including some used for chemotherapy, are also made from plants, but in modern medicine, they tend to be purified in the lab. Another characteristic of ethnodrugs, is that their preparation and use, is based on traditions developed over thousands of years, during which they've been tested. Our drugs, on the other hand, are based on controlled clinical experimentation, and scientific medical knowledge, biochemistry and pharmacology. Our drugs are based on scientific research while ethnomedicine is based on experience gained over years of tradition. Ethnodrugs can sometimes be useful, and in certain cases, such as that of PSK, they outweigh the scientific filters, and give us elements to produce drugs or dietary supplements. In any case, the most important contribution that ethnomedicine can give us when treating diseases such as cancer, is a lesson about method, about approach, about our philosophy of care.

Ethnodrugs mirror a different way of thinking than our medicine does. Knowledge about remedies has been gained over long periods of time, and through trial and error. There is no scientific research to discover the remedies and give relative security. This method requires risk taking, having the courage to deal with the bad and going ahead in uncertainty. Traditional treatments are also less aggressive: they don't try to eliminate the cause of the illness, but rather try to restore the natural balance that has been broken, so that the individual can live rather well, even if the illness is still there. Being able to live with the bad, and having courage, are just the things which are needed in order give up conventional chemotherapy use, and begin to try to control the cancer by other means, pushing off chemotherapy as time goes by.

Why do oncologists tend to use chemotherapy poorly?

For the most part, oncologists think that there are essentially two really effective treatments: surgery, and chemotherapy. The first is used when the cancer is found early, before it has become metastatic. The other, chemotherapy, is currently thought of by oncologists as the only real weapon that we have in fighting metastatic cancer. Oncologists habitually undervalue other tools which apparently don't work as well as chemotherapy, but which can in any case be helpful in keeping cancer under control, or at least slowing it down, especially when used together, in combinations.

Precisely because they rely exclusively, or nearly so on chemotherapy, oncologist tend to fall into a downward spiral. When they see signs of metastatic cancer, they do chemo. If they don't see a response, they do another chemotherapy as soon as possible. If there is a response, they think that the only thing to do is to wait, because they only believe in chemo, and it's not a good idea to repeat it without a valid reason. After some time, the disease inevitably recurs, and the stakes are raised. At each successive chemo, the cancer cells become more resistant and aggressive. As a consequence, chemo really does become the only weapon available, and stronger and stronger chemotherapy treatments are needed.

To avoid falling into this downward spiral, oncologists should try with all available means to keep the cancer under control for as long as possible, before it becomes aggressive and resistant. That's what Leonard does while treating Helen. The first chemotherapy had been inevitable, because of how serious the illness had become, it was threatening Helen's life. After the success of the chemotherapy, Leonard does everything possible to keep in control of the cancer without striking it with a second chemo. Each time that the illness comes back, he searches for a way to deal with it without using chemotherapy, sometimes by adding new remedies that help to slow the cancer down, without bothering Helen too much.

REALISM, PROACTIVITY, AND MULTIMODALITY: BEHAVIORS TO DEVELOP

In order not to fall into the downward spiral of repeated chemotherapy treatments, realism is needed. We need to objectively eva-

◆◆◆

95

luate the effectiveness of chemotherapy, and realize that as effective as it may be, chemotherapy can never completely eradicate cancer. Oncologists sometimes put too much stock in it, it could be that they sometimes lose sight of the goal of helping the patient live a long and healthy life, and behave as though their mission was to try to obtain a momentary success with chemotherapy. It's a typical human error, concentrating on the immediate consequences of our choices, without stopping to think about our trajectory.

It's also important to be proactive, to be able to foresee future developments, and act preemptively. Only by being proactive are we able to work at keeping control of the cancer before it reappears, pushing off having to do another chemotherapy. Leonard is being proactive when he worries about the little button which reappeared in the stomach, and it is thanks to his proactiveness that Helen can avoid undergoing a second chemotherapy treatment at the standard interval of less than a year.

Having a multimodal approach, as apposed to a monomodal one, means relying on multiple solutions at the same time, instead of only on one. Oncologists fall into the chemo spiral, also because they tend to have a monomodal way of thinking, as if the treatment has to be based on only one method that they really believe in, chemotherapy. Monomodal thinking, for the most part, also characterizes scientific research, which experiments with one medicine at a time. Clinical research, or at least part of it, is still Galilean, it still uses Galileo Galilei's way of doing research. The fundamental principle of the Galilean method is to simplify reality, remove some of the many factors involved, and focus on just a few. But if we really want to try keeping in control of cancer, we need to use multiple remedies at the same time, each one might not do much on its own, but used together, they can help us to obtain our goals.

The art of being a tamer

Try to imagine leaving your house and finding a lion in your yard, maybe a runaway from the zoo. It's there in front of you, it stares at you. What would you do? You don't have the weapons to kill it, nor do you have a way to capture it. You definitely can't challenge it, seeing as that it wouldn't take much for the lion to kill you. In order to have any chance at all, you must unsheathe the art of being a tamer.

You stay calm, and without letting him know it, you control every detail, hoping to anticipate his every move. You use all of the signals available (your posture, your voice, the way you look at him, etc.) so that the lion also stays calm. You would do anything to make sure that he stays calm.

If we really want to manage a metastatic cancer, we need to un-sheathe the art of being a tamer, just as if we had a lion in front of us. In the case of the lion, we can always hope that someone will come and save us, or that somehow, we will be able to get away or go back in the house. With cancer though, that isn't possible. Realistically, only death from other causes can liberate us completely from cancer.

Metronomic chemotherapy: a good resource for the tamer

From the moment that the little button appeared in her stomach, Helen went ahead with metronomic chemotherapy. This is a kind of treatment that has been gaining in popularity over recent years. It consists of taking low doses of chemotherapy, usually orally, with continuity, or better put, without long breaks. Helen took 4 capsules of UFT a day, 5 days a week. A metronomic treatment using 50 mg of cyclophosphamide a day, is common. Combining 50 mg of cyclophosphamide daily with 5 mg of methotrexate given as a twice weekly pill, or with capecitabine are also commonly used. Sometimes capsules of vinorelbine are given three times a week, with doses that vary from 30 to 50 mg for each dose. In cerebral tumors such as gliomas, temozolomide, which unlike many other drugs is able to reach the brain, is used.

Metronomic regimes vary, but low doses and continuous administration is common to them all. To understand how low these doses are, we have only to think about a standard chemotherapy using cyclophosphamide, these are given together with other chemotherapy drugs, at doses of around 200 mg a day given orally, or at doses of around 1000-2000 mg every three weeks intravenously. Researchers talk about LDM chemotherapy (low-dose metronomic), compared with MTD chemotherapy (maximum tolerated dose), seeing as how in standard chemotherapy, doctors try to raise the doses but keep them just below the limit where they become intolerable.

Metronomic chemotherapy is well tolerated, even though there sometimes are side effects, and at times problems can be seen as the treatment goes forward in time. For example, when using cyclophosphamide, doses should never exceed a total of 25-30 grams (500-600 days, with 50 mg a day), because there is the risk that if we surpass this limit, the accumulated toxicity can cause leukemia. Metronomic chemotherapy has the enormous advantage of not spoiling the patient's life, given that it's usually done by taking capsules or pills comfortably at home.

It's an interesting fact that cancer cells have difficulty becoming resistant to metronomic treatments. It used to be believed that there weren't any resistances. We now know that these are possible, even though they are quite rare. In any case, what happens with chemotherapy doesn't occur: that we find ourselves passing from one line to the next, with a progressively lower chance of success. On the contrary, changing the type of metronomic treatment is a good thing, because it confuses the cancer cells. These cells become accustomed to a specific drug, and are in trouble if the drug is changed. Pasquier, Kavallaris and André have named this the drug-driven dependency/deprivation effect or 4D effect.

Metronomic chemotherapy doesn't pull us into a spiral like chemotherapy does, it doesn't lower the patient's quality of life, nor does it expose them to the serious risks of a standard chemotherapy. However, it doesn't have give us the same results as a successful chemotherapy. Cases with brilliant responses to metronomic therapy aren't lacking, and when evaluated with standard criteria, as used with chemotherapy, it's relatively effective in the bigger picture. For example, with metastatic mammary cancer, clinical studies using metronomic therapy have had response rates that ranges between 12 and 88%. With weekly docetaxel, one of the most widely used chemotherapy drugs, the response rate are between 30 and 68%.

These results at a first glance seem comparable, aside for the fact that the metronomic results seem to vary more widely. The response rates include both total as well as partial responses, and with weekly docetaxel, we see higher percentages of complete response. Metronomic treatments on the other hand, tend to give more partial responses and stabilization of the illness, results which frequently aren't included in the response rates.

In any case, we shouldn't expect too much from metronomic therapy. The best way to use it is to help keep in control of the tumor, to tame it, and gain precious time before the next chemotherapy.

Metronomic and conventional chemotherapy

Differently from conventional chemotherapy, metronomic chemotherapy is comfortable and well tolerated. If used correctly, it doesn't cause serious risks, and doesn't pull us into a downward spiral. To compensate, it works better as a way of keeping in control of the cancer, than in attacking it head on. Metronomic chemotherapy allows us to use trench warfare, rather than go on the offensive. We can better understand why this is if we explain how metronomic therapy works.

Standard chemotherapy kills neoplastic cells. Metronomic chemotherapy usually doesn't kill them, but rather makes their lives difficult. In order to grow, tumors need blood vessels, and so they produce these vessels through a process called angiogenesis. Metronomic treatments inhibit angiogenesis, and force the cancer cells to live with fewer blood vessels.

Another effect of metronomic chemotherapy is that it enhances immuno-surveillance, the control mechanisms that our immune system uses against the neoplastic cells. Through these mechanisms, reducing the number of blood vessels that the tumor has available to it, and strengthening the organism's immune defenses, metronomic therapy pushes the tumor into a state of rest. In a certain sense, it puts the tumor to sleep, even though it doesn't kill it.

HOW METRONOMIC THERAPY WORKS

Metronomic therapy slows down tumor growth through three main mechanisms, which create unfavorable conditions for the neoplastic cells and make them less active.

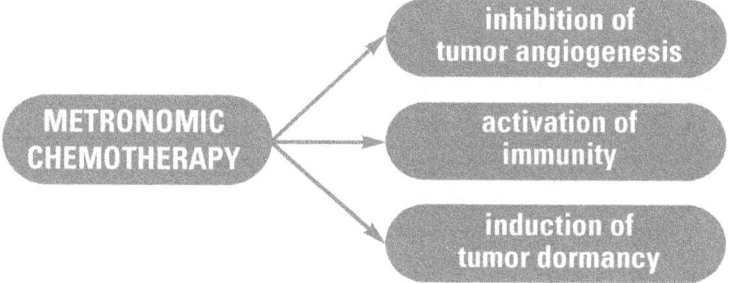

Angiogenesis is the production of new blood vessels. This makes it possible for the tumor to receive sufficient oxygen and nutritional substances for growth and to dispose of waste. Metronomic therapy inhibits angiogenesis in multiple ways. It acts on endothelial cells which form the new vessels, it reduces their availability and blocks their proliferation and migration. It increases thrombospondin 1, a molecule which is able to inhibit angiogenesis.

One way that cancer cells escape from the immune system's attack is through the action of regulatory T cells, cells which suppress the activity of lymphocytes which would be able to kill (CD8 and NK). Metronomic therapy increases the lymphocytes which kill cancer cells, reduces regulatory T cells and reduces the immunosuppressive activity that these cells have.

◆◆◆

Metronomic therapy pushes cancer cells into an inactive state, like sleep. It does this because it inhibits angiogenesis and so reduces the availability of oxygen and nutrients, it starves the cells. It also puts the cancer cells to sleep by stimulating immunity, so it induces them to be inactive to escape the immune system's cells. It also uses direct methods, such as arresting their proliferation, to put the cancer cells to sleep.

Another mechanism is sometimes added to these three main ones: The 4D effect (Drug-Driven Dependency/Deprivation). Metronomic therapy is a treatment which is continual. In the long run, the cancer cells become dependent on the particular environmental conditions which are produced by the metronomic drug. Suspending the metronomic therapy or changing drug can throw the cancer cells in crisis by removing the drug which they had become accustomed to.

The 4D effect makes metronomic therapy particularly interesting. The interruptions which are done in order to recover from the side effects, which although modest, exist, can increase the success of the treatment. Alternating different drugs can be helpful for bearing the treatment, and at the same time, it can make it a more effective treatment.

Mistaken ideas about metronomic chemotherapy

Metronomic therapy is clearly completely different from standard chemotherapy. In both cases we use chemotherapy drugs, but because they are used in a different way, their action against the tumor is completely different. This explains why a drug can work well with metronomic treatments, even with a cancer that has become resistant to the same drug used in a standard manner.

Sometimes oncologists fail to fully understand how different metronomic and traditional chemotherapy really are. For example, they are reluctant to use a metronomic treatment with vinorelbine in a patient who was unresponsive to a vinorelbine based chemotherapy. They seem not to understand the fact that a tumor can be resistant to vinorelbine when administered with traditional methods, but not when administered in a metronomic manner. The action mechanism for each of the two therapies is completely different.

A similar thing happens when oncologists ask themselves whether the drug to be used in the metronomic therapy has a high success rate for the type of cancer being treated. They are thinking in the same way that they would think about a traditional chemotherapy treatment, without giving enough importance to the fact that it is a completely different treatment.

When using traditional chemotherapy, each cancer has specific drugs which are more or less recommended for that specific cancer type. With metronomic chemotherapy, the choice of drug isn't rigidly based on the cancer type. Even though clinical experience and reasoning guides us in our choice of drug, in theory, we could use the same drugs for different tumor types. It's easy to understand the reason why, if you understand that the drug given with metronomic chemotherapy doesn't kill the neoplastic cells. There aren't cells which are more or less receptive to a specific drug. Metronomic treatments work indirectly, creating difficult conditions for a tumor, any tumor, to grow in.

When Leonard decides to add UFT to the tamoxifen, the remote second opinion disappoints him, because the doctor says that there is no proof that UFT is effective against metastatic breast cancer. It is as if the doctor doesn't understand that Leonard plans on using the UFT in a metronomic manner, and so it makes little sense to ask ourselves about the effectiveness of the drug in Helen's type of cancer. The decision should be based on other considerations, like tolerability, or the fact that it has been tested in combination with the other drugs that are being used. Based on these considerations, Leonard thinks that it would be a good idea to combine UFT, tamoxifen and PSK.

Why don't oncologists take advantage of the potentials of metronomic therapy?

Oncologist frequently use metronomic chemotherapy as a last resort, as an extreme attempt when the standard treatments have all failed. At other times it is used with elderly patients, or those in poor condition. They take advantage of the fact that metronomic therapy is well tolerated and doesn't compromise the quality of the patient's life. On the other hand, they are willing to accept the modest results that it offers, because they no longer have any hope left for a successful treatment, or because they don't want to overburden the patient.

Using metronomic therapies in this way makes sense, but limiting ourselves in this way means to under-use this type of treatment. Oncologists who limit themselves to using metronomic treatments in extreme situations makes the mistake of considering it in the same way they consider standard treatments, as a weapon of assault. They don't realize that it's most important use is for trench warfare, during the time that we need to hold on, and keep the cancer at bay. For example, oncologists rarely think of using metronomic therapies after a successful chemotherapy. Why should we keep still without doing anything, when the tumor has regressed? Isn't this the precise moment to start with a less aggressive treatment that puts the cancer cells to sleep and which could help to delay the next chemotherapy treatment for some time?

Metabolic modulation: a challenge that should be accepted

When the illness comes back to the stomach for the second time, Leonard substitutes lansoprazole with ranitidine and adds octreotide. These are two simple moves which give surprising, though short-term, results. They work by modifying the gastric environment, making it more hostile to the cancer.

Previously, when they were dealing with the problem of diarrhea caused by the UFT, Leonard had introduced zinc carnosine with the intention of protecting the intestinal mucosa. He had felt sure in his choice also because he had thought that zinc carnosine

103

could contribute to making the gastric environment less favorable for the cancer's growth.

Years later, seeing the markers rise, Leonard avoids chemotherapy simply by changing the hormone therapy. This change is based on the discovery that the stomach produces estrogens which are capable of stimulating the tumor's growth, and aims to make the stomach less rich in estrogen.

These therapeutic interventions that Leonard uses are examples of metabolic modulation, biological changes with specific aims, which work to push the cancer into a corner. Metabolic modulation is difficult. On the one hand, care must be taken not to cause damage to the organism: the strategies that we use need to be well tolerated. On the other hand, it's quite a challenge to analyze all of the intricate biochemical pathways which we are working with, and to calculate all of the effects of our modifications. To get a good idea about these challenges, it's enough to look at the endocrine environment chart that Leonard built when deciding whether to change the hormonal treatment (see page 68). It puts together a series of information to be built upon: the stomach is able to produce androgens (androstenedione e testosterone), starting with cholesterol and circulating progesterone, these androgens are then transformed into estrogens (estradiole) by aromatase which is present in the stomach's parietal cells, and in the cancerous cells.

It isn't easy to find means, drugs or food supplements, which can produce the changes which we are trying for. It's important to study, read up on things and carefully examine all of the various possibilities. There are many options, but they are usually overlooked. It's a good idea to start with the analysis of the specific case, to try to understand the kind of environment the cancer cells find themselves in and what can be done to make it less favorable. Creativity must be mixed with scientific rigor.

Even though metabolic modulation is challenging, it still is worthwhile to try. It sometimes, like in Helen's case, gives us surprising results. This is possible because cancer cells adapt themselves to the environment which they live in, so changes in this environment can make things very difficult for them, at least until they find alternative strategies of adaptation. In other cases, metabolic modulation doesn't give immediately evident responses. In any case, it can sometimes be helpful in keeping the cancer under control, and supporting other strategies. It is an additional resource for the tamer.

The promise of biological therapies

In recent years, biological therapies have been cause for hope. They are called biological therapies because they either use substances taken from living organisms, or synthetic compounds which mimic actions of molecules present in our bodies.

BRMs such as the PSK that Leonard uses are considered biological therapies, along with other treatments which work to strengthen the organism's defenses. The hopes of recent years, are mostly tied to molecular targeted therapies, which target specific molecules present in cancer cells, thereby inhibiting their growth, or killing them.

Molecular target therapies without a doubt are useful, but the hopes that they have aroused might be excessive. Some of them cause serious side effects, and they can sometimes be very expensive. Others are better tolerated and have lower or at least more accessible costs. None of them though, cause miraculous effects, nor are any of them remedies that can completely resolve the problem at hand. They are only helpful when used wisely.

One reason that molecular target therapies can't completely resolve the problem, is that cancer cells are able to adapt very rapidly. When we act on certain molecules, blocking specific biological activities necessary for the survival of the cancer cells, these cells find alternative ways to grow and thrive. Bevacizumab, for example is a very successful drug, which has proven useful especially when used together with chemotherapy or radiotherapy. It works against VEGF, which is a proangiogenic factor, in this way helping the cancer. VEGF stimulates the production of new blood vessels which the cancer cells need in order to thrive. A problem with using bevacizumab is that over time cancer cells become resistant and spread elsewhere in the body. Recent studies demonstrate that when the inhibition of VEGF gives the cancer cells problems, these cells adapt themselves to produce new vessels even though the VEGF is blocked, or they migrate to other areas.

In theory, molecular target treatments could be resolutive if we find ways to block all of the possible biological pathways which the cancer cells could use to survive and to grow. For the moment though, this remains a dream. It's a good idea to accept biological treatments for what they are, a resource among many that can help tame the cancer, slowing down its development for as long as it's able. Since some of them are toxic, as well as expensive, it's important to carefully analyze the costs and benefits.

Leonard was at times, tempted to use bevacizumab or trastuzumab, which act on HER2 receptors, which then interact with estrogen receptors. His calculations of the costs and benefits though, dissuaded him: in Helen's case, all things considered, it didn't make sense to use these drugs at the time, but rather to save them for possible future use.

The temptation of invasive surgery

When Stephen T. considers the hypothesis of surgically removing the stomach, Leonard doesn't agree. In the end, Helen goes with the method of keeping the illness under control using a combination of systemic therapies and locoregional treatments. Leonard thinks that removing the stomach would mean condemning Helen to an unpleasant lifestyle, and in any case, even after removing the stomach, the disease would almost certainly reappear.

In later years, Helen and Leonard have often reflected about the idea of removing the stomach, especially when things didn't seem to be going well. They asked themselves, "Who knows if things could have worked out better?". The disease was present only in the stomach and getting rid of it by removing this organ was an attractive idea. But later on, when looking back, Helen and Leonard realize that not having removed the stomach had been a wise choice.

Helen used to say, "Imagine if I had to live with metastases elsewhere, and moreover without my stomach". Leonard wondered, "So many years have passed, and you've been doing so well. Who can guaranty that we would have been given all this time had we removed the stomach? We may have gained more time or maybe less. In any case the quality of life would have been worse". Of course some doubts still lurked in the back of their minds, because when dealing with cancer, we have to make decisions without being sure. We can only try to make informed and reasonable decisions.

Surgery can be an attractive option when treating oligometastatic cancer, that is cancer with metastasis in one or only a few parts of the body. Interesting studies done using significant numbers of patients suggest that for certain types of cancer in specific sights, surgically removing the metastasis can prolong the patient's life, sometimes by quite a lot. It is a good idea though to be careful, to carefully weigh out the pros and cons of the treatment, just as Helen and Leonard did. When deciding, we must always keep in mind the idea that surgical removal, even if it it could work in our specific case, can never completely put an end to the disease. For this reason it is best not to overestimate the benefits, or underestimate the possible harm that it could cause.

Minimally invasive locoregional treatments

In Helen's case, the metastasis which appeared in the stomach had been previously treated with mucosectomy combined with photodynamic therapy and later with repeated cryoablations. At a certain point, Leonard considered using intratumoral injections of chemotherapy drugs and metabolic modulators, between one cryoablation and the next. These are all minimally invasive locoregional treatments which can be used in the stomach. They are easily done with endoscopic procedures, similar to a simple gastroscopy.

Minimally invasive locoregional treatments can be a wonderful tool when taming cancer, when trying to keep it at bay and gain time. They have the advantage of being usually well tolerated, and can frequently be done as outpatients, without hospitalization. Another important advantage, is that they work by destroying the tumor while causing minimal or no harm to the patient. Complications are always possible, just as with any treatment, but these are rare, especially if the treatment has been carefully chosen, paying attention to the site, and all likely risks.

Minimally invasive locoregional treatments should be used early, as soon as metastasis is seen in any part of the body. It's easier to treat metastasis when it is still confined to a small area, it is less risky, and causes less damage. We see better results, also thanks to the fact that by acting sooner, we can gain more time through the treatments. The cleanse should be done as soon as possible.

Even though it's fairly clear that locoregional treatments should be done early, we frequently make the mistake of waiting too long and deciding too late. There are some oncologists who aren't great fans of minimally invasive locoregional treatments. Some sustain that there isn't enough scientific evidence demonstrating their usefulness, this isn't actually true, seeing as how significant evidence has been accumulating over time. For the most part, oncologists prefer to trust in invasive surgeries and chemotherapy, and not in minimally invasive locoregional treatments, with similar attitudes that they have for metronomic therapies. They tend to use these treatments only when in a state of crisis, and they are at a loss for what to do next. This is a bad use of locoregional treatments, which just like metronomic therapies, give their best results when played ahead of the game, acting against metastasis as soon as it is noticed, and trying to prevent the cancer from escaping from our control. Helen's case, as seen from this point of view, is emblematic.

It is sometimes thought that locoregional treatments should be used only once. Edward B. had been disappointed that the disease had returned even after the mucosectomy, and the photodinamic therapy. He wasn't expecting Leonard to ask him to continue treating the cancer in the stomach, and he certainly never expected to do dozens of treatments.

It's best to start with the idea that the illness will almost certainly be back after the first treatments: this is the nature of cancer, it is a chronic illness. The situation, and the tools at our disposal don't always permit us to repeat the treatments. Leonard had carefully studied the situation before finding ways to repeatedly treat the stomach metastasis. When possible, after having found the right way, it is always a good idea to be ready to repeat the locoregional treatments. Helen got it right when she said, "If you sweep every day, your house will stay clean".

Unfortunately, it isn't easy finding your way among the many locoregional treatments available to us. At times, even oncologists aren't completely well informed about them: they are familiar with some of them, but ignore others, in yet other cases, they don't even know which hospitals perform certain treatments. This is partly because, along with well known standard treatments, there are others which haven't been well documented or well experimented on. They may be uses in one specialized center or another, but information about them doesn't circulate in the scientific and medical community. Paradoxically, sometimes less well known treatments that aren't standardized are the most interesting ones.

If an oncologist tells us that no minimally invasive locoregional treatments exist for our specific case, we shouldn't blindly believe them. We should ask them to go and study all the possibilities, with care and patience.

Personalization of care: a dream
that must become reality

We usually talk of personalized medicine, to mean the use of tailored drugs, based on genetic or biomolecular analysis. Oncologists already do this in many cases. For example, in mammary cancer, hormone therapy is used when there are estrogen receptors. But as Leonard had discovered to his surprise, only the alpha receptors are analyzed, and not the beta receptors. In any case, decisions are made based on molecular analysis.

At other times, personalized use of drugs is recommended, even if it isn't commonly used. We know for example that tamoxifen works well for women who have a genetic type with an active CYP2D6 enzyme, an enzyme which transforms the tamoxifen into its more active metabolites, 4-hydroxytamoxifen and endoxifen. For this reason, there are those who recommend other types of hormone therapies to women who don't have that genotype. Frequently though, these preliminary examinations and these targeted therapeutic decisions aren't done, mostly for practical reasons. Not even Leonard had Helen do these tests, both because the scientific evidence was still unclear, and because it wasn't practical to have these tests done in a short enough time period to be useful.

Some people put a lot of hope in a tailored medicine, based on genetics and molecular research. We will probably go further with these techniques in the future, but this kind of personalized care is expensive and complex.

We can also think of personalized care in the more general sense of guiding therapeutic decisions based on the person, their lifestyle, and specific features of their disease. In oncology, this kind of personalization should be the goal, but frequently it isn't applied. Frequently, we end up following protocols or guidelines that tell us how to treat one class of oncological illness or another. As hard as we may try to carefully classify oncological diseases, we will inevitably regroup different patients with different diseases and medical histories, treating them all in the same way.

If we start to accept the point of view of personalization in cancer care, we will see that each case is different, and that the same case is at each moment a new case, in the sense that it changes during the history of the disease. This becomes evident if we think about Helen's story. The diffuse visceral metastatic cancer of the beginning of the story, is completely different from the small button that appeared in the stomach later on. The situation is once again completely different when the illness comes back aggressively in the stomach, and it continues to change as time goes on. Over time, the cancer cells changed in a variety of ways. Leonard was able to stay on top of some of these changes, but a great many, probably the majority, escaped his notice. The gastric environment, the metabolism, and the body's defence mechanisms also changed over the course of the story.

If we really want to manage the illness, gain time, and live well, we must realize that the cancer care has to be extensively personalized. The situation should be analyzed, using all of the information available, on a moment by moment basis. We must consider all possible therapeutic options, and make our decisions as the need comes up, paying attention to all of the factors at play. This is a very difficult and complicated job, but perhaps it is about time that we started doing it.

Why is it that oncologists so rarely personalize treatments?

Personalizing is very difficult. Leonard dedicated himself to the personalized care of only one person, Helen. Oncologists usually are treating multiple people, with different types of cancer, at the same time.

Personalization also calls for bravery. To really do it, we need to be ready to discard standard treatments, and adventure along new, and sometimes unbeaten paths. Helen and Leonard's story is eloquent. Who had ever heard of doing all of those cryoablations in the stomach? Where was the clinical testing, the evidence, the guidelines to tell us how to proceed? Repeated cryoablations apart, Helen's care differed from standard conventions at almost every step. Guidelines recommend to wait and then, when the progression is evident, change hormonal therapy or perform a new chemotherapy. Leonard though, decided to add UFT and PSK to the tamoxifen, without waiting, and so on.

The doctor who gave them her remote second opinion scolds Leonard in one of her letters, asking him why he is conducting an almost experimental treatment. After much consideration, Leonard realizes that the doctor is right, but he doesn't understand why it is so scandalous to use an almost experimental treatment. In any case, for a doctor who is treating a stranger, deciding to use an almost experimental treatment it is a test of courage. Sometimes doctors have to work with state laws that regulate the use of certain drugs, setting strict circumstances for their use. If things don't go well, there can also be the risk that their work can be put under accusations by the patient or his loved ones. Of course, if the doctor has an in depth discussion with the patient and his family, and they reach an agreement, the doctor and patient can rise to the challenge of personalizing the care, knowledgeably. To do this though, we need oncologists who are also good psychologists.

There is another reason why doctors tend to personalize so rarely, which may be less evident, but is no less important. In order to take on the burden of personalized care, the doctor has to have a firm belief that it is useful. As long as we continue to search for treatments to resolve the illness once and for all, simply using chemotherapy and surgery, we won't understand why we have to take on the burden of personalized care. Only those who grasp that the way the illness is managed makes the difference are willing to personalize the care.

It is important to be careful about the decisions which are taken at each step and the philosophy of care.

The error of "wait and see", and the art of knowing how to wait while meanwhile planning in advance

The rule as it is usually practiced of waiting and watching is not a good rule. While we are watching and waiting, the metastatic cancer starts to come back, and we will soon find it back in full force even stronger than before. A patient shouldn't be left without treatment between one chemotherapy and another. Helen has never stopped taking medicines or doing local treatments which keep her cancer at bay.

It's also important to monitor the illness carefully, and catch the first possible signs that could help us know what should be done to slow it down. We should plan ahead whenever possible. This is exactly what Leonard does when he has the gastroscopy performed earlier than planned, as soon as he sees the CEA rising, thus discovering the little button in the stomach, and adds UFT and PSK to the tamoxifen.

If on the one hand it's true that we should always stay ahead of the game, it is also true that on the other hand it's important to know how to wait.

Different signals can cause us to worry that the illness is spiraling out of control during the time that we are holding it back with mild treatments. After many cryotherapy treatments Leonard saw the CEA and CA 72-4 rear up, and Stephen T. thought of going back to chemotherapy. Leonard studied and pondered to try to find a way to curb the cancer without going back to using chemotherapy. He found good reasons to limit themselves to only changing the hormonal therapy. That is what he did, and it worked well.

His decision hadn't been easy. There was always the risk that the cancer could slip out of their control. It's important to keep a delicate balance between being proactive and being patient. Managing to get the balance right is a real art, achieved through careful study of the case, analytical reasoning, and above all, self control.

Long life to cancer

Helen, when she is in a good mood, calls her cancer "my brother cancer", meaning that at this point they live together, they are inseparable. She has accepted the fact that cancer is a chronic illness, and that the goal when treating it should be to be able to live well for as long as possible, to carry on with life even though you have cancer inside of your body.

She is well aware of the fact -having thoroughly discussed it with Leonard- that metastatic breast cancer is aggressive. She can't reasonably hope that it behaves like some thyroid cancers, which are only discovered at the autopsies of people who died of other causes. It's likely that it will be just her own cancer which kills her in the end, but she hopes that it leaves her time enough to live, and preferably to live well.

Helen says "my brother cancer" with a touch of irony. She thinks of a paradox which she finds very funny. The treatments aren't able to kill the cancer. The chemotherapy is limited to killing a certain number of cancer cells, but the cancer survives. Even when there is a complete remission, such as in her case, there are still some cells, even if only a few, which can't be seen with the methods that are at our disposal.It is from these cells that the cancer restarts. Leonard has explained to her that in the quest to eradicate cancer, some high dosage chemotherapy treatments have been tested, along with bone marrow transplants, to try to save the patient. Even these strategies have ended up failing. "They are like monsters in a science-fiction film -says a smiling Helen- they fall to the ground under machine gun fire, and then get back up again rising from the flames when we thought they had been burned alive".

So, even with our current capabilities, the only way to kill cancer is by killing the host, the person inside of which it is developing and growing . For this reason, if this is really the way things are, it makes sense to wish a long life to the cancer. "If my cancer is alive -Helen explains to those who ask her- it means that I am alive. This is the reason that I wish it a long life, and that I really consider it as a brother. After all there are also unpleasant brothers". The paradox which she finds so funny, lies in the fact that she is wishing a long life to something which is probably going to be the cause of her death.

Beware of the error of determinism

After a long time that the illness in the stomach is being well managed, Stephen T., who was worried about the rising markers, writes to Leonard saying that he thinks the time has come to use chemotherapy again, he observes, "Many years have passed, we should be satisfied". He seems to think that they should use chemo, because normally a metastatic breast cancer doesn't remain quiet as long as in Helen's case.

When his relative who is a pathologist praises Leonard's work, he shows him the latest survival statistics of metastatic breast cancer, that he has just received. It seems as though his way of reasoning is: you're doing a great job, because according to the statistics Helen should already be dead.

Stephen T.'s way of thinking, and that of the pathologist relative, are spoiled by the error of determinism, a well known error, which frequently causes us to misunderstand scientific acquisitions. This error consists in thinking that if scientific research has discovered a rule of some kind, or a scientific law as we sometimes call them, this means that things will definitely go according to that rule. John Kemeny, a philosopher of science, explains this mistake clearly,"The law is not in any case something binding, rather it is a simple description of all events, past, present, and future". So the survival statistics for metastatic mammary cancer are just a description of how things usually go. It is a mistake to think that just because that is what the statistics say, that is how things will definitely go in my specific case. This would mean confusing a simple description of facts, with the mechanism which causes them to occur.

Helen intelligently notes, "The treatments are part of our life, and we don't live within the statistics, on the contrary, it is the statistics that mirror our lives". For his part, Leonard thinks that they're fighting against the cancer, not against the statistics. What is important to him is that Helen lives long and well, not that they beat the statistics.

The error of determinism dangerously creeps into the minds of cancer patients and their families, as well as in the oncologist's minds. A doctor can decide, as Stephen T. was willing to do, that it's time to act, just because too much time has gone by according to the statistics. He can become satisfied with the achieved results, and possibly even fight less because the statistics are comforting. Even if the patient has a progression, doesn't respond to treatment, and dies, the overall treatment can be looked at as a success, because the survival is in the right quintile, in the 20% of those who have survived the longest.

Cancer patients who know these statistics sometimes think that their time has run out, they succumb to fear, become resigned and ready to surrender. We should remember that taking statistics as a binding law is a logical error, we should concentrate on fighting our own personal battle.

Be careful not to make a myth out of science and medicine

Basing care on scientific knowledge is fundamental. Leonard avidly explores scientific literature, searching for useful information. This information sometimes gives him ideas and suggestions for possible treatments, sometimes it helps him to carefully evaluate his decisions, to put them to the test of the most severe criticism. Science has its limits though, it is far from being an oracle, capable of providing us with the answers to all of our problems. The accumulated knowledge of modern biological science and of medicine is extraordinarily advanced and vast. But if we think about problems such as cancer, we must admit that even though we have gained a great deal of understanding, we actually know quite little. Newton said that a scientist is like a child who analyzes the shells on the shore of the great and boundless sea. Our knowledge of seashells is useful, but we have yet to discover the great and boundless sea.

It is also important to note that scientific knowledge evolves, and that with scientific progress, what we believed yesterday to be true, may seem false today. Leonard comes across the problem of scientific progress when he thinks about adding UFT to the tamoxifen. The opinion at a distance strongly tells him that hormonal drugs (like tamoxifen), and chemotherapy drugs (such as UFT) shouldn't be associated with each other. This principle has been surpassed, it is based on scientific reports that scientific research has revised later. Leonard knows this, but the doctor of the second opinion has remained anchored to doubts of a science which is already old.

Keeping the limits of science clear helps us to understand one point: scientific knowledge is extremely useful, but it can not be a substitute for the oncologist's intelligence. Oncologists can't simply be people who apply what science says. They, when confronted with a given case, must think, and make a synthesis of what we know and of what we don't know. They must evaluate certainties, uncertainties and probabilities, and take responsibility.

Medicine is a practice which stands on the shoulders of medical science. Like other practices, it is organized, with structures and routines. The connection between medical science, and medical practice is far from obvious. In order to base their work on medical science, doctors would have to constantly read scientific literature, studying each time in order to respond to questions that the cases elicit, or to find knowledge that could be useful to them in some other way. They would also need to consult with each other about cases that they treat, and make use of special software which give them immediate access to helpful information. Traditionally though, doctors tend to base their treatments on things that they already know, that they learned while they were studying or updating themselves. They don't always have an intense study period for each case that they're treating, like Leonard did when caring for Helen.

Seeing as how medicine isn't science, but practice which is based on science, there is always the risk that it might become a simple implementation of protocols. When researchers do a clinical trial, they test a protocol, which is a precise pattern, with certain features of the disease, patient, treatment and follow-up. Doctors who are caring for a patient sometimes merely repeat already tested protocols which are well known in science. In oncology, this happens frequently because the pathology is serious, and the treatments challenging, also psychologically. Oncologists can find refuge in protocols. However things end up going, they can say, both to themselves and others that they used a tested and consolidated protocol.

Unfortunately, simply applying protocols means not taking a personalized approach to care. A protocol is designed for a category of people with the same illness, not for the specific person that the doctor is treating. What they should focus on is that person. Thinking about the specific case, and the specific conditions would help them better treat the disease. It is appropriate to consider the protocols. However, oncologists must also ask themselves what is the rationale for their choices, that is, on what information, scientific knowledge and reasoning these are based. Leonard for example, bases his decision to change hormone therapies on a rationale that comes to him after he discovers that the stomach produces estrogen, and that is made clear in the elaborate graph that he built together with Helen (see page 68).

We shouldn't turn science and medicine into myths. We must remember that they can be extraordinary resources, but we must also remember that they have their limits. So politely make sure that your oncologist doesn't just implement a protocol, but that he is dedicated to studying about your case, even by consulting with other experts. Also make sure that he uses his own intelligence in order to carefully consider what he has learned from studying about your case. We shouldn't trust a doctor who gives us the impression that things seem obvious to him. Battling with cancer is never obvious, for anyone.

Why is it that oncologists at a certain point either become decisionist, or give up?

This usually happens when things aren't going well. It can happen from the beginning, if the cancer is, like in Helen's case, serious from the start. In the famous center where Leonard and Helen went at the beginning of story, the specialist surrenders in front of what he believes to be an advanced ovarian cancer. He takes Leonard aside, and says that in his opinion, it may not be worth it to try chemotherapy. In the same situation, another oncologist might have had the opposite reaction and tried everything, playing the card of a reckless therapy.

Giving up, or being decisionist are behaviors which are frequently seen later in the story of the care after many failed attempts based on standard strategies or ones that had been carefully thought out. In these last cases, the fact that the oncologist put so much effort into the treatment causes him to think that some special action is needed, or that there is nothing left to do. With a closer look though, we see that these ideas are mistaken, because the effort that we put into something is not a good way to measure the validity of that action: the fact that we worked very hard doesn't necessarily mean that we worked well, we might have been working hard on the wrong things.

Decisionism and resignation partially mirror the tendency to consider cancer as an acute disease. If an illness is acute, it has to end in one way or another. So either we find treatments effective enough or we surrender. Our way of thinking is different if we accept the idea that cancer is a chronic illness. In that case, we don't need to see signs that the illness is retreating, it's enough to know

119

that it isn't advancing to much, that it remains calm enough to let us live in peace. From this perspective, decisionism and resignation don't make much sense, because the important thing is resisting.

The error of determinism can contribute to decisionism and resignation. An oncologist can be influenced by the statistical probability of being able to successfully treat a serious illness or one that has been going along for a long time. In Helen's case, the specialist of the famous center which they had consulted in the beginning of the story, had apparently calculated the probability of being successful and was pessimistic, also because he mistakenly thought that the cancer was in the ovaries. Stephen T. recommends chemotherapy at a certain point because the idea of a metastatic mammary cancer that has gone along for so long, even without chemotherapy, is strange to him.

Sometimes decisionism and resignation are tied to a psychological uneasiness that an oncologist may feel because of his experience with his medical profession. These are ways of safeguarding his psychological integrity, even if he continues to have to deal with failure. When he is resigned, the oncologist is playing the part of the one who looks coldly at reality, who knows that nature can be hard, and who is able to leave behind the feelings which would like nature to be different from what it is. When he is decisionist, he challenges nature, he reclaims his human sentiments, and feels completely human, even if in the end, it is the disease who wins.

The oncologist's burnout

Oncologists are subject to burnout, a psychological syndrome which people in helping professions, especially health care, are exposed to. Among health care professionals, oncologists are among those with the highest risk of burnout.

As the word suggests the person suffering from this syndrome is burned out, exhausted. Those who are burned out feel as if they no longer have the resources to relate to people and help them. In order to deal with these feelings, they react in various ways: sometimes they are cold and distant, at other times they are sullen, or they follow rules to the last detail like a bureaucrat, or are afraid of making mistakes or of being misjudged, they are in a state of alarm.

There are many factors invoked to explain burnout in professionals such as oncologists. The fundamental cause seems to be the imbalance between the investment that the professional makes, and the feedback that they receive, that is signals which tell them if their work has been useful or not. A professional like an oncologist frequently starts out driven by ideals, thinking that his work is a mission, which will help others and turn him into a benefactor. As time passes though, he receives many signals that tell him that this isn't the case, and in the long run he gets burned out. The signals which burn out oncologists are mostly the many patients that he looses despite his best efforts to care for them.

Burnout can contribute to certain questionable behaviors of oncologists, such as using excessively aggressive treatments, not accepting the fact that cancer is chronic, following protocols too rigidly, not personalizing the treatments enough, and giving up, or being decisionist. If we sometimes notice that an oncologist is elusive, not focused enough on relationships, or a bit cynical or in crisis, it could be that he is suffering from burnout.

Realizing that oncologists can suffer from burnout can help us understand our own oncologist and manage our relationship with him in a way that works well for us. When we see certain questionable or unpleasant behaviors, we shouldn't stiffen up. We should try to help him find in himself the momentum that he needs to be able to seriously try to treat us better.

The oncologist's best interest, and the patient's best interest

The best interest of the patient, and that of the oncologist converge, but they don't always completely coincide with each other.

The patient wants to deal with the illness, cancer, which is afflicting him, and the oncologist wants to treat him. But what exactly is the goal that each of them set for themselves?

Helen and Leonard frequently don't follow the specialists' recommendations, because their goals are different from those of the specialists. In their story, the difference are mostly about their philosophy of care, the way that they think about cancer and cancer care. Differently from some experts whom they consult with, Helen and Leonard think that cancer is a chronic illness, that the important thing is keeping it under control not eliminating it, that chemotherapy is an extreme weapon, and that non-aggressive treatments and minimally invasive locoregional treatments should be taken seriously, that the patient's care should be highly personalized.

Sometimes the oncologist's best interests and the patient's don't coincide because the oncologist is mostly worried about managing his commitment and feeling all right about himself. So he finds refuge in protocols and established practices. Instead, a careful and courageous personalization can be better for the patient. In certain moments, the oncologist's main interest may be to manage the psychological discomfort of his burnout, taking care of his professional disease. The patient is obviously more concerned with treating his cancer.

When discussing our care with an oncologist, we should try to understand what his interests are, and if they really coincide with our own. Oncologists frequently concentrate on the diagnosis and on the therapeutic options available in that kind of cancer, maybe analyzing the possible results. We shouldn't content ourselves with this. We should explore their philosophy of care point by point, and ask polite, yet precise, questions. We should check to see if certain choices respond to his psychological needs. Sometimes to check, it is sufficient just to observe the other person while they are speaking, or see how they react to simple innocent questions, "Why should we go with this therapy regimen?", "Are there any other options?", "Wouldn't it be best to further study my case?", "What happens if my treatment doesn't work?", "How will I be feeling during my treatment?", "Are we sure that it wouldn't be better to use a less aggressive method?".

The technique of 3A for talking with oncologists

If we try to understand the oncologist's interests and compare them with ours, it may happen that we find out that our viewpoints are different. What should we do in such a case? How should we manage the dialog with our oncologist?

When we discover that we have a different vision in a specific matter than the person whom we are talking to we frequently make an effort to be accommodating so as to avoid tension. It is enough to be less rigid, less sure of ourselves, and less firm in our judgments, make the effort to bring our point of view closer to that of the other and find common ground. When talking with our oncologist, it isn't a good idea to use this strategy of everyday life. The stakes are too high, these different points of view are all about our care, and at the end of the day, about our lives. This isn't something to be accommodating about. We should be trying to understand what is actually best for us. This quest to understand is too important to give up in the name of peace and quite.

Because the stakes are so high, you might think that it's a good idea to openly confront your position with the oncologist's. Sometimes, in certain situations, it can be beneficial to do this, but in general, it is a bad idea.

In response, oncologists sometimes take a trench warfare position: they tell us or lead us to believe that their way is how things are done and that it's not possible to do otherwise. After all, they are the experts. Instead of being entrenched, the oncologist could give up and align himself with our position without debate, after all, we are the ones with the problem, and it really is a very important problem. If you think about it, neither of these cases are ideal. We end up doing one thing or the other, without having sufficient dialog or exploring the options together. One person ends up imposing themselves, and the other person gives in. In reality, the important thing isn't establishing who is in command, and who must obey. Once again, there is too much at stake for things to go this way. There is also the fact that the relationship is troubled to some extent. We will have much less serenity in a relationship that is so important to us at this stage of our life.

So what should we do? It can be helpful to learn the rule of the 3A. The first thing to do is take what the oncologist proposes seriously. Listen carefully to what he says, point by point. This is the first A, Attend, be interested and listen.

With this approach, we then pass on to consider things and to reason together with him. We should do this seriously. His viewpoint becomes our own, we must really get into it and think like he does. Assess, carefully consider, justify and think over.

At the end, we arrive at the third A, Address, orientate our counterpart within reality. We should talk about our concerns, about what we would like to see happen, our desires. We don't do this to contrast our ideas with the oncologist's, but only to remind him that we exist and that we see things in this way. We should make sure that it's clear to the oncologist that these aren't objections to his ideas, which are great, but rather a way of telling him who we are and what we are thinking. We are helping him to orientate himself in the world, since there are not only diagnosis, treatment and clinical reasoning, but we are here and it is our life which is at stake.

It is important to complete all three of these steps. Otherwise this technique doesn't work, and we fall back into the conflicting points of view with trench warfare behaviors, or become condescending. If the oncologist, after hearing us present ourselves, with our thoughts, hopes and desires, continues to repeat his point of view, we just start with the first A again, and then move on to the second and then the third. It is a circular motion which could theoretically repeat itself infinitely, but it usually stops after a few cycles.

When using the 3A, we make the issues clear and get to the bottom of the problems. At the same time, we don't sacrifice bringing our own viewpoints to the forefront, and avoid conflict in our relationship with our oncologist.

DO THE 3A WHILE DISCUSSING WITH THE ONCOLOGIST

An example may help us understand the 3A. The oncologist proposes aggressive therapy. The patient is more inclined to be less aggressive. He manages the oncologist politely, by doing the 3A.

Attend
– We are thinking of doing eight cycles of docetaxel and gemcitabine.
– Why is that?
– Even though we only see the one metastasis in the liver, the illness is probably widely spread. It's a good idea to go with a treatment which cleans things up.
– That makes sense.

Assess
– It's an association that has a high success rate.
– Let's hope that it also kills the cancer cells that we can't see.
– That's what we're hoping. We'd like to reset the illness. That's why we're thinking of doing even more cycles.
– That would really be great!
– Oh yes!

Address
– What worries me though is the idea of putting myself through chemotherapy like that for just one lump in the liver. I would feel better if we first tried to remove the lump in some other way, maybe with a non-aggressive treatment.

MINIMALLY INVASIVE LOCOREGIONAL TREATMENTS

TECHNIQUE	WHERE IT IS USED	NOTES
Radiofrequency or RFA (radiofrequency ablation)	liver, bone, lung, kidney, brain, parathyroids, esophagus, stomach, retroperitoneal masses	A needle is inserted into the tumor. An electric charge is then passed through the needle into the tumor, which is destroyed. It is useful for pain in bones, and can be combined with cementoplasty in order to consolidate bones. In hollow organs (esophagus and stomach) it should be avoided, because of the risk of perforation. There are other techniques which are preferable for the brain.
Cryotherapy or cryoablation or cryosurgery	liver, lung, kidney, prostate, esophagus, stomach, skin, breast	Substances able to freeze are put in contact with the tumor, either directly or with needles that penetrate the skin or with laparoscopy, endoscopy or bronchoscopy. This treatment is safe and well tolerated. With skin and mammary cancers, the treatment can be painful.
PDT (photodynamic therapy)	esophagus, stomach, lung, bile ducts, pancreas, peritoneum, ovaries, mouth, larynx, bladder, prostate, brain, skin	A light sensitive substance (usually Photofrin or ALA) is administered systemically. The tumor is then illuminated with an appropriate light and is destroyed. It is necessary to wait for a period of time between treatments, especially when using Photofrin. After the treatment, it is important to avoid light exposure.
Laser therapy	skin, uterus, vagina, vulva, penis, lung, trachea, esophagus, stomach, colon, brain	There are multiple types of lasers, but in general they are lights with specific wavelengths. They are strong and precise like a scalpel, and can destroy tumors. The lase-

TECHNIQUE	WHERE IT IS USED	NOTES
		r's precision is particularly useful in situations such as brain surgery where it is important not to damage the tissue surrounding the tumor in order not to worsen the patient's quality of life.
Alcoholization	liver, thyroid, pancreas	High concentrations of alcohol (> 50%),when injected into a tumor, provoke necrosis and destroy the tumor. If the injected alcohol goes outside of the tumor, there is a risk of complication. For this reason, alcoholization should be avoided in organs, such as the stomach and lungs, where diffusion is likely to occur. In these organs, it is possible to use alcohol in lower concentrations (up to 5%) together with chemotherapy drugs. At low concentrations, alcohol strengthens the effectiveness of chemotherapy drugs without causing necrosis.
Intratumoral chemotherapy	in all easily reachable sites	Intratumoral injections take advantage of the fact that it's possible to reach concentrations inside the tumor that are higher than would be possible using the same doses systemically. For this reason, it is possible to achieve the desired effect while at the same time reducing side effects. The chemotherapeutic concentrations remain high for only a short period after the injection. For this reason, slow releasing formulations have been made, although these have the disadvantage of exposing the organism to the chemotherapy drugs

TECHNIQUE	WHERE IT IS USED	NOTES
		for longer periods of time thus increasing the possibility of side effects. When these drugs are injected into hollow organs such as the esophagus, the stomach, or the colon, because of the risk of perforation, it's important to use drugs that can't provoke local damage.
Intra-arterial chemotherapy	liver, pancreas, stomach, eye, mouth, head, brain, lung	This method consists of injecting chemotherapy drugs into the arteries which bring blood to the tumor, in a very well aimed fashion. It gives us the advantage of flooding the tumor with the drug, while at the same time reducing the quantity that is found in the rest of the organism. This reduces toxicity. It is important to remember that even though at this time, the techniques are refined and commonly used, reaching an artery with a catheter is a very delicate operation. On a case by case basis, it's a good idea to do a cost-benefit analysis.
Chemoembolization	liver, other sites	Anticancer drugs are injected into the arteries that serve the tumor, together with embolization particles which close the small vessels trapping the chemotherapy drugs, and remove oxygen and nutritional factors from the tumor. This treatment is followed by a post-embolization syndrome and can have complications.
Minimally invasive surgery	abdominal organs, spinal cord	With minimally invasive surgery it is possible to operate without creating large openings in the body to access the organ. Using laparo-

TECHNIQUE	WHERE IT IS USED	NOTES
		scopy in the abdomen for example or in the digestive tract with endoscopy. This keeps the damage to a minimum. The treatment can sometimes be an outpatient procedure, and is generally well tolerated. The use of robots makes minimally invasive surgery safer and more effective. Some surgeons are still attached to using traditional surgery techniques even when minimally invasive ones are available and might be better indicated. They think that when dealing with cancer, it is best to remove as much as possible. They, for example prefer to remove the whole stomach even if the tumor is circumscribed. This is an error, because if the tumor is well circumscribed, minimally invasive techniques are equally effective and make it possible to have a better quality of life.
Radiotherapy	multiple sites	Radiotherapy usually tends to cause significant damage in the area around the tumor. In a smaller measure, this is also true for the so called radiosurgery, a more specific type of radiotherapy. Before undergoing radiotherapy, it is always a good idea to see if there are any more selective methods of treatment. For example, in cases of cerebral lesions of a small size, it would be a better choice to use lasertherapy which spares the healthy part of the brain making it less likely that brain damage will give us unwanted effects.

A SMALL DICTIONARY

Ascites This word is used to indicate an accumulation of fluid in the abdominal cavity. This fluid can be more or less abundant, and either only be visible with echography or other tests, or it can give us evident symptoms such as heaviness and bloating. In most cases, ascites is caused by diseases of the liver, usually cirrhosis, which causes an increase of pressure in the veins which bring blood to the liver from the digestive tract and from other abdominal organs, and causes a transudation of liquid into the cavity. It is more rarely caused by cardiac problems, or by the fact that the peritoneum (see peritoneum) produces an exudate, an inflammatory liquid. It can also be caused by illnesses, among which are gastrointestinal tumors, or tumors of other abdominal organs or by a peritoneal carcinomatosis (see peritoneal carcinomatosis).

Biopsy This is the removal of a tissue fragment for analysis. It is performed with different methods depending on the site. In the stomach, it is done with gastroscopy (see gastroscopy).

CT scan A radiological exam which permits us to obtain detailed images of different parts of the body, thanks to the fact that the signals gathered by the scanner are then elaborated on a computer with specific algorithms. CT is the abbreviation of computerized tomography.

Cytoplasm The part of the cell which is surrounded by the membrane and which surrounds the nucleus (see nucleus). It is made of a base structure, the cytosol, where the organelles (particular structures with specific functions) are found.

Electrolytes Chemical elements, with either positive or negative electric charge, which are found in the blood and the rest of the body. They are particularly important for successful functioning of the cells and the organism. Sodium, potassium, chlorine, magnesium, and calcium are normally measured in the blood.

EUS Endoscopic Ultra-Sonography, is an echography done in digestive endoscopy, through a probe which is inserted in the mouth or anus. Echography is an imaging diagnostic technique which is based on the fact that different tissues absorb the echos from the ultrasounds, in different ways. EUS makes it possible to examine the wall of the digestive tract and other organs in the vicinity such as the pancreas and bile ducts.

Gastrectomy A surgery to remove all the stomach (total gastrectomy) or a part of the stomach (partial gastrectomy).

Gastroscopy A technique for examining the esophagus, the stomach, and the duodenum. It makes use of a probe with a camera attached to it. It is inserted through the mouth.

Hypersensitivity reactions These are immune reactions to substances which are foreign to the organism, they have damaging effects instead of defensive and beneficial ones. Four different types of reactions are distinguished.

Imaging diagnostics Also called imaging, is the act of producing images of internal parts of the body with specific techniques. These techniques include echography (see EUS), traditional radiography, CT (see CT), magnetic resonance imaging (see magnetic resonance imaging), PET-CT scan (see PET-CT scan).

Magnetic resonance imaging Also called nuclear magnetic resonance imaging, or simply resonance (or MRI). It is a imaging diagnostics technique (see imaging diagnostics) which takes advantage of the rotation of nuclei produced by their exposition to a magnetic field. Like the CT scan (see CT scan), it is a morphological exam, which differs from the PET-CT scan which is capable of giving metabolic and functional information.

Mammography An radiography of the breast, to find neoplastic formations. It is habitually used for breast cancer screening.

Neoplastic cachexia Is a syndrome connected to tumors, and characterized by a loss of appetite, weight loss, loss of muscle mass, weakness, anemia, and worsening general conditions. Neoplastic cachexia is mentioned, as opposed to non neoplastic forms of cachexia which are caused by other diseases.

Nucleus A formation which is usually highly visibly inside of the cellular cytoplasm (see cytoplasm). It contains chromosomes, and has the function of conserving the genetic information and guiding the cellular activity.

Oximeter An instrument which makes it possible to measure the frequency and intensity of the pulse and to estimate oxygen saturation levels, the amount of oxygen in the blood. It uses a probe, usually tongs which are applied to the finger. It is usually connected to an electrocardiograph, and a graph can be continually viewed on a screen. With the oximeter, the principle vital signs which are indicators of the organisms functioning are always under control.

Peritoneal carcinomatosis (or carcinosis) Is the infiltration of the peritoneum (see peritoneum) by the cancer, usually with the presence of nodules and ascitis (see ascites) and with tumoral cells in the ascitic fluid.

Peritoneum A thin membrane which covers the abdominal cavity and the organs which it contains.

PET-CT scan A diagnostic imaging exam (see diagnostic imaging), in which a CT scan (see CT scan) and a PET scan (positron emission tomography), a technique of nuclear medicine which makes a scan of positrons emitted by radioactive substances injected into the body, are performed almost simultaneously. In oncology, glucose which contains radioactive fluoride, 18FDG (Fluoro–Deoxy-Glucose) is used. The neoplastic areas are seen, because cancer cells attract glucose, so they pick up more 18FDG than healthy cells. The CT scan permits the localization of areas with abnormal uptake. Differently from CT scans (see CT scans) and magnetic resonance imaging (see magnetic resonance imaging), the PET scan is a functional test, and not simply morphological, this sometimes makes it safer for the identification of neoplastic areas.

Vital signs See oximeter.

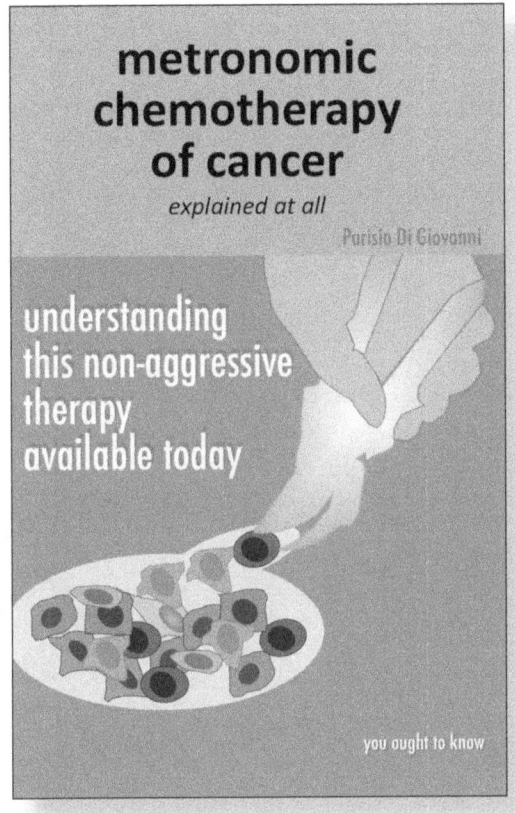